Also by Jay McGraw

Life Strategies for Teens
Closing the Gap

The Ultimate Weight Solution for Teens

The 7 Keys to Weight Freedom

Jay McGraw

Free Press

New York   London   Toronto   Sydney

Names and identifying characteristics of people in this book have been changed.

This publication contains the opinions and ideas of its author. It is intended to provide helpful and informative material on the subjects addressed in the publication. It is sold with the understanding that the author and publisher are not engaged in rendering medical, health, or any other kind of personal professional services in the book. The reader should consult his or her medical, health or other competent professional before adopting any of the suggestions in this book or drawing inferences from it.

The authors and publisher specifically disclaim all responsibility for any liability, loss or risk, personal or otherwise, which is incurred as a consequence, directly or indirectly, of the use and application of any of the contents of this book.

FREE PRESS
A Division of Simon & Schuster, Inc.
1230 Avenue of the Americas
New York, NY 10020

Copyright © 2003 by Jay McGraw
All rights reserved,
including the right of reproduction
in whole or in part in any form.

First Free Press trade paperback edition 2003

FREE PRESS and colophon are trademarks
of Simon & Schuster, Inc.

Designed by Charles Kreloff

For information regarding special discounts for bulk purchases,
please contact Simon & Schuster Special Sales at 1-800-456-6798
or business@simonandschuster.com.

Manufactured in the United States of America

10   9   8   7   6   5   4   3   2   1

Library of Congress Cataloging-in-Publication Data is available.

ISBN 0-7432-5747-2

I dedicate this book to my best friend, my brother Jordan

And to:

Mom
Dad
Amy
and
Grandma

With Very Special Thanks to:

Jan
Shannon
Frank
Maggie
Leah
Scooter
Anthony
&
The Free Press team
Dominick
Suzanne

And to:

All of you who have shared with me your stories;
your willingness to share will change the lives of many.

Contents

An Open Letter to Parents from Dr. Phil

Dear Parents,

My opening words in the original *The Ultimate Weight Solution* were: "You have a decision to make." For my readers, that decision involved whether to stop chasing after fad diets and start making the right choices to take lasting control of their weight. That was their decision.

But as parents, reading these words, you have a different decision to make. This one has to do with your children and whether you will decide to become a genuinely positive influence on them at a pivotally important period in their lives.

Here is the problem: Kids today are getting fatter and more unhealthy right before our eyes. More than 30 percent of our children are overweight, and more than 15 percent are obese. Anorexia, bulimia, and other eating disorders have gone vertical.

These heartbreaking problems—childhood obesity and eating disorders—are out-of-control epidemics, like a train careening at an ever-increasing speed down a steep hill. If you're a parent reading this, that means you may have a kid on that train whose life could very well be heading toward a tragic wreck.

I not only believe that this train can be stopped, I know it can be stopped. One of the most important vehicles to stopping it is you.

Let me explain: Your children do not have the ability to predict the consequences of their actions and therefore cannot be expected to make reasonable and mature decisions about food, weight, or dieting. They do not have enough information about what certain choices and eating habits may create in their lives.

But as parents, we have that information. We know so much more than we did even a generation ago. We know that the revolution in computer technology has created a generation of kids who are computer potatoes. We know that fast food restaurants are being built on every corner of our neighborhoods, and worse, infiltrating our schools, selling and perhaps addicting our kids to obesity-promoting foods. We know that if our children become obese, then they are likely to stay obese throughout most of their adult years. And we know that with obesity comes heart disease, diabetes, cancer, and other diseases that can and do kill.

You must use that knowledge to parent your children in a way that keeps them from abusing food in an unhealthy manner or risking an eating disorder to look the way they think they want to look.

I have no doubt that many of you at this very moment are thinking that you don't know where to start, that maybe you tried before and you don't feel like starting again. But I can tell you that what you have in your hands right now is a good starting place and a new beginning—this book, written by my older son, Jay. I have been humbled and proud over the gift he has to reach out and communicate to teens everywhere. Now he has used that gift to talk to teens who are troubled over their weight, their bodies, and really, their self-esteem.

Jay did a tremendous amount of research to prepare for this book, from conducting a survey of 10,000 teenagers to interviewing professionals in the weight and psychological fields to reading everything he could get his hands on that talked about adolescent obesity and eating disorders. Then he wrote it all down, translating the 7 keys of the adult version in such a way that teens can "get" and incorporate in their own lives. Inside this book are solutions that work, whether your teen's challenges are obesity, body image problems, or an eating disorder. If your kids read this book and do its work, they will tap into the power to create meaningful change and start living with a healthy regard for themselves.

But it takes more than a book. It takes you.

Always remember that your children rely on the role models in their lives—and that's you. So hold up the mirror to look at yourself. You will see that whatever your kids are doing, you may be modeling the very same behavior—and with it, setting your children up for success or for failure.

What I'm asking you to do is hold yourself to a higher standard. I am asking you to be someone for your children who sets the right example and inspires your children to rise to a new, nobler level. Expose them to healthy kinds of food. Create a lifestyle for them that includes regular exercise. Model healthy choices. Encourage and uplift them in a way that protects their health and enhances their self-esteem. Through your actions, your words, and your love, direct your children toward where you want them to go and all that you want them to be.

You can help build an extraordinary life for your children. Don't let them down. Setting an inspiring, loving example can be the single most significant act of your life, and the greatest gift you can give your children.

Dr. Phil McGraw

Introduction

Viewing Options: ➡ view all messages ➡ view all messages ➡ outline view

UNTITLED MESSAGE

Hi, my name is Alison and I am SOOOO sick of being the fattest girl in my class! I am 5 feet 2 inches tall and I weigh 211 pounds. I hate it and I hate being me. I have always been fat, and I feel like it is not my fault, but I have no idea what to do about it.

➡ reply to this message ➡ add to favorites ➡ view all replies

Viewing Options: ➡ view all messages ➡ view all messages ➡ outline view

UNTITLED MESSAGE

My name is Gina, and I am 14 years old. I weigh 180 pounds, and I am really interested in this guy at school. My weight has never really been an issue to me, but now that I am interested in guys, I hate being fat. My friend is so skinny and so beautiful, and I just want to be like her. I cry myself to sleep at night, because I just want to be different, but I don't know what to do. I am even thinking about throwing up after I eat. I figure that will probably make me thinner.

➡ reply to this message ➡ add to favorites ➡ view all replies

Viewing Options: ➡ view all messages ➡ view all messages ➡ outline view

UNTITLED MESSAGE

I always hide in my bedroom and just bawl my eyes out because I am always the fattest one. Every time we go anywhere no one even acknowledges that I exist. I know they see me because I am so big, but they just ignore me. Would someone please tell me how to lose weight?! I am desperate. I feel like a horrible person, but I really just have no idea what to do. Please help me!

➡reply to this message ➡add to favorites ➡view all replies

Viewing Options: ➡view all messages ➡view all messages ➡outline view

UNTITLED MESSAGE

I have been throwing up my food for almost a year now, trying to be skinny. It's working, but I'm afraid that I'm going to hurt myself. I'm scared that my mom is going to find out, but at the same time I want someone to catch me. I can't stop, but I need to. Would someone please help me?!

➡reply to this message ➡add to favorites ➡view all replies

Viewing Options: ➡view all messages ➡view all messages ➡outline view

UNTITLED MESSAGE

I'm on the cheerleading team, and I love it, but I'm constantly worried that I'm going to gain too much weight and get kicked off of the team. I'm always dieting. I just want to eat cake at my friends' birthday parties, but I hate myself if I do. Even when I do diet, I still don't lose any weight. I really wish someone would tell me what to do and how to do it. It seems weird that everyone loves my body except me. How can I be the only person at school that thinks I am fat?

➡reply to this message ➡add to favorites ➡view all replies

What's up? I'm Jay McGraw, and what you just read are examples of some typical web postings. Since you're reading this book, I'm guessing you relate, at least in some way, to what the people above have to say about their weight, their bodies, and their appearance.

Maybe you feel like they do. You want to lose weight. You want to feel better about your body and the way you look. You want some control over your life.

But you probably don't have any idea what to do about it. Well, I have some good news. Actually, I have some great news. By picking up this book, you've finally found the answer. This book you're holding in your hands is one of the most complete and accurate answers you will ever have for figuring out how to get yourself in shape—and without being obsessive about it.

As a young person, I know how hard it is to get people to take us seriously and give us the information we want and need. So I decided to find the information myself. I did a huge amount of homework for this book—more than I've ever done before, because I know how important is to all of us to finally have a real, serious answer. With this book, I'm giving you exactly that.

So, that means it is time for you to take a deep breath and get ready, because starting right now, you have the information you need to learn to accept yourself and get the body you've always wanted. As you make your way through this book, you will learn there are seven keys to a healthy mindset and a body you are proud of. At times, the process will be fun; other times it will be tough. But no matter what, if you read, understand, and apply these seven keys, I promise you, the result will be worth it. This plan will work—but only if you commit yourself to following it.

You're about to start feeling good in your body and feeling good about your body. With the solutions you'll learn and put into action in this book, you'll get more freedom and more control over food, your weight, your body, and your entire life than you can ever imagine. Just count on it!

Excited? Great. Me too. I'm going to be there with you the whole way. Right about now you're probably thinking "Who are you?"

Fair enough. I am a 24-year-old law student at Southern Methodist University in Dallas. Before law school, I got an undergrad degree in psychology from the University of Texas and wrote two other books for teens—and before that, well, I was in high school just like you are now. I make no claims to be a therapist. I'll leave that to my dad (You know him better as Dr. Phil, the guy with the talk show, but you can just think of him as "Jay's dad.")

And speaking of research, I put together a team, including doctors, nutritionists, and psychologists to advise me about what's in this book. I read every scientific article I could on teen weight issues (and you thought Shakespeare was bor-ring!). I also designed and conducted a survey that was supervised by the Department of Rehabilitation, Social Work, and Addictions at the University of North Texas, in Denton, Texas, one of the best departments in the nation in terms of eating disorders and related addictions.

In the survey, I questioned more than 10,000 teens on how they feel about weight and food—plus tallied up the results myself. With these results, all of the articles that I have read, and the info I gathered from my team, I feel very confident that I know what you need to learn from this book.

Okay—so why did I write this book, anyway? I wrote it because I've talked to thousands of teens all over the country about what's going on in their lives. And I know that weight issues are a big deal with teens. I know that a lot of you are feeling pretty bad about yourselves because you think you're fat or unattractive. I want to help you change that, but not just on the outside. That's a tiny part of it. I want to help you change on the inside so you can learn to love yourself and treat yourself better.

If you want to know more about me, check out www.Jay McGraw.com or www.DrPhil.com. Both of these websites will tell you a lot about who I am and what I do.

Get psyched, because you are about to begin one of the most life-changing experiences you'll ever have. Let's go!

An Important Message to Parents

According to a recent study published in *Pediatrics,* the journal of the American Academy of Pediatrics (AAP), if you have a child or teen who follows a restrictive diet, your child may actually gain more weight over the long term, compared to other young people who do not go on diets. In their study of boys and girls ages 9 to 14, researchers reported that restrictive diets are hard to stay on and can lead to binge eating and cycles of jumping back and forth between dieting and overeating—all factors that could be responsible for the weight gain. The study suggests that a better approach, if you have an overweight child, is to encourage changes in lifestyle, including regular exercise, and to stay away from any diet that severely restricts calories. This book provides guidelines and strategies to help teens avoid extremes—and as a result, help them make healthy, positive changes in their weight and in their lives.

This book will do two things for you as parents. First, I not only outline the healthy lifestyle that this study talks about, but perhaps more important, I tell you how to implement it into a busy teenage life. Second, this book has been written for teens; what you as parents can learn from that is how to talk to teens about this topic. It is virtually impossible to teach someone something when they don't understand what you are saying and why you are teaching them. This book solves that problem for you. *The Ultimate Weight Solution for Teens* is written in a way that teens understand the material presented. If you as parents read this, you will then be able to communicate the material to them in a way that they see the value in your message. This book will allow you to create a plan and a lifestyle that is safe, healthy, and effective both now and in the long term.

The Ultimate Weight Solution for Teens

Chapter 1

The Solution You've Been Looking For

G et ready. You are about to learn the best teen strategies for taking control of your weight and getting in better shape.

This book is for teens who want to manage their weight and get in shape—but without resorting to crash diets or trying to get thin thighs in two weeks.

When you get finished reading this book, and putting its steps into play, you will look and feel so much better about yourself. You will reach that point of satisfaction with your body where you will no longer be embarrassed or ashamed of yourself, or obsessed with your weight, or self-conscious about your butt or your belly.

But let me be real honest with you right up front: Not all teens need to lose weight. You may be at a healthy weight already, and so losing weight is something you shouldn't do.

But a lot of teens try to lose weight when they don't need to, or they go on a diet for all the wrong reasons. You do it because you think people will like you more, or because all your friends are doing it. You do it to fit in. Or you try to lose weight because you think you're not as thin as you'd like to be. Or maybe your parents are pressuring you to lose weight. Losing weight sounds like something you should be doing.

But losing weight may be unhealthy for you. Instead of trying to take pounds off because everyone else is doing it or because your parents say so, it is a good idea to check with your doctor to see if you have too much fat on your body for your age and height.

This is really important. If you find out that you need to drop some pounds, great. Getting in better shape can be a good thing. But make sure you're doing it because you need to—and for the right reasons. Don't do it for your boyfriend or girlfriend. Don't do it to fit in. Don't do it for your parents. Do it for you.

That's what I will help you with on every page of this book: how to do it for you and how to do it right.

You and Food

Here's the first thing you have to realize about your weight—it's not really about a number on the scale or a size on the label of your Levi's. It's about whether you use food to take care of your body or abuse it and do just the opposite. Maybe you never thought about food like this. Here are some examples of what I'm talking about.

Using food to take care of your body	Abusing food and hurting your body
Eating good foods	Eating too much junk food
Eating when you feel naturally hungry	Bingeing on food
Not going on guilt trips over what you eat	Throwing up food on purpose
Not going on diets	Going on extreme diets

Abusing food causes problems. The most common one is being overweight. We're spending too much time at Mickey D's and not enough exercising. In your head you know it's not worth it. Feeling like a big blob is a frustrating and depressing way to live. Meet Melissa, a 16-year-old high school sophomore who admits she abuses food and has battled her weight all of her life because of it. She once shared with me what it feels like to live in this dimension:

Viewing Options: ➡ view all messages ➡ view all messages ➡ outline view

UNTITLED MESSAGE

I've always been what you'd call a "fat girl." Nobody's ever really made fun of me, at least not to my face, but people do treat me differently. Guys don't think I'm pretty, so I never get asked out. Girls who are smaller than me avoid me, and I feel even bigger and uncomfortable around them. Sometimes I feel like the cute, small girls are a totally different species from me. The few friends I have are big like me, and we don't even go out much. It's kinda like we're grounded, not by our parents but by our own bodies for being fat and too embarrassed to be seen. When things go wrong, I head for candy and cookies. Pretending that life is okay doesn't take the sting out of the shame I feel over my size. I cry a lot. I'm disgusted with my body and with myself because I can't lose weight, and I think about suicide almost every day. I really do. I've never been happy with myself, and I hate my life. I've always felt that if I was thin, life would be so much better.

➡ reply to this message ➡ add to favorites ➡ view all replies

Melissa is like a lot of teens. She's unhappy with her body. She's unhappy with herself. She feels like her life is a mess. Her bad feelings are setting her up for trouble. If you share some of Melissa's characteristics, you're not alone. About a third of all teens are overweight. Being overweight brings on teasing from people that messes with your head. It causes a lot of emotional pain, period. When all you want to do is wear a belly-shirt like Britney Spears, and you can't, every single day feels like the end of the world.

But I'm here to tell you that being overweight doesn't make you a loser or a freak. This book will help you get real about yourself and your body. It will help you change some ideas you have about yourself. It will help you and the Melissas of this world live the best that's within you.

Eating Disorders: Dying to Be Thin

Being overweight isn't the only problem. Some of you may be dealing with eating disorders. Two of the most common are anorexia, a kind of self-starvation; and bulimia—that's when someone eats ungodly amounts of food (bingeing), then gets rid of it by throwing up or taking laxatives (two forms of "purging").

Eating disorders are not just about food or weight. They're attempts to deal with insecurities, sadness, stress, and problems with family and friends. This is serious stuff. If you think you've got a problem in this area, stay with me throughout this book, but definitely check out Chapter 11. It's written just for you.

The first time I heard about an eating disorder, long before I researched the subject, was when I was in high school. Here is what happened.

From kindergarten on, Pam and I were best buds. Pam was always a really pretty girl. She wasn't just cheerleader material—she *was* a cheerleader *and* homecoming queen. But that's not the only thing I appreciated about Pam. As we got older and started high school, what I really came to like and respect about Pam was her intelligence. She was so smart. I mean, she read *Catcher in the Rye* just because she wanted to before it was ever assigned in English class, and she took physics even though she could have stopped at chemistry and had *no* science her senior year. (Now admittedly, at the time I couldn't decide if this made her smarter or dumber because my definition of smart was always to do as little schoolwork as possible. But looking back, I'd say Pam is and was a practical genius.) I used to have her help me with my algebra (this was before you could get *Algebra for Dummies* on CD-ROM). I needed help because I was sort of average—a C student, at best, during my first two years in high school before I smartened up and graduated with honors. I wasn't in the top half of my class. I guess I was the one who made the top half possible!

One day Pam was supposed to come over and help me figure out how to find the square of an algebraic sum (which I never did figure out). I was up in my room waiting for Pam when my mom came to my room and said, "Pam's not coming over; she's in the hospital."

In the hospital! I automatically thought she must have had a car accident or hurt herself at cheerleading practice. Scenarios of stitches and broken bones raced through my head. I never would have imagined anything else. Pam was healthy, energetic—she was a cheerleader, for goodness' sake!

Well, it was none of the above. Pam was rushed to the emergency room because her mother found her throwing up blood in the bathroom. Nobody knew until that moment that Pam was suffering from bulimia, and had been since seventh grade. It was this huge secret that she lived with every day for years, and now it had landed her in the hospital hooked up to IVs and machines. She almost died!

As it turned out, the whole ordeal was a blessing because it got Pam on the road to recovery. Much later, she poured her story out to me, and I want to share part of it with you.

Viewing Options: ➡view all messages ➡view all messages ➡outline view

UNTITLED MESSAGE

All I ever thought about was being skinny. My friends and I would constantly talk about carbs, and calories, and fat, and about 98 diets, and being thin. I was terrified of getting fat. If I gained even a pound, I felt horrible, so I was always on a diet. When I lost weight, I felt really good and in control, like I had achieved something. But sometimes I'd eat more than I meant to, and I'd feel really bad about it. One of my friends told me about purging. I was willing to do anything to be thin, so I I tried it. Then I started doing it more and more. Sometimes I'd throw up ten times a day. I got so good at it that all I had to do was manipulate my stomach muscles and the food would come up. I didn't care if I was hurting myself. I wouldn't stop. I couldn't stop. I got really good at hiding it so that I wouldn't have to stop. I hated myself for it, but there seemed to be no way out.

➡reply to this message ➡add to favorites ➡view all replies

Pam felt stuck. She thought that she was in a place or a situation that she couldn't get out of. She was doing what she was doing because it is all she knew how to do, but eventually, Pam found a way out, and so can you. Whatever form it takes, using food in unhealthy ways can sink you into a deep hole, and the longer you stay in it, the harder it will be to get out. This book can help you pull yourself out. I want you to start feeling good about yourself—and not be so hung up on your appearance.

The Seven Keys to Weight Freedom

Whether you're wrestling with being overweight, trying to climb your way out of the deep, dark hole of an eating disorder, or just want to develop a healthier attitude toward food and your body, I'll give you a special set of tools—they're called keys—to help you solve these problems, once and for all.

What are these keys? Well, there are seven of them, and they are based on another book, one that my dad wrote, the original *The Ultimate Weight Solution—The 7 Keys to Weight Loss Freedom*. My dad's been a psychologist since long before any of us were even born, and he's counseled thousands of overweight men and women, and people with eating disorders. The seven keys are what he's used to help all those people. Dad says that these seven keys are what you need to lose weight and take care of your body. They're not some new fad diet, either. They're a way to help you change the way you look at yourself, and just as important, the way you treat yourself. And that's the kind of change I know you're looking for.

Okay, I'm sure you're wondering what these keys are all about, so let's get to it. Here they are, followed by a super-brief explanation.

Key 1: Right Thinking
Success from the inside.

Key 2: Healing Feelings
The end of eating emotionally, purging, or doing other unhealthy things to your body.

Key 3: A No-Fail Environment
Cruise control for getting fit.

Key 4: Mastery Over Food and Impulse Eating
Get it together: no more bad food habits.

Key 5: Jay's Portion Power Plan
Warning: This is no-diet territory.

Key 6: Intentional Exercise
The fun factor in fitness.

Key 7: Your Circle of Support
Friends are for helping—and keeping you accountable.

So there they are—the seven keys to freedom from food issues. Let me tell you something up front: The seven keys are not a get-a-better-body-in-two-weeks program. As Bart Simpson once wrote a hundred times on the chalkboard, "I will not sell miracle cures."

And I won't.

But when you use these keys in your life, you'll have an instant edge—you'll look, feel, and live better—for real. Other people might not notice an immediate difference, but you will! And what's better is that the results will last. The keys are just the tools you need to do it.

If I had to sum up the seven keys in a few words, they'd be: simple, doable, and totally powerful. But the best part about the seven keys is that there is no willpower required!

No Willpower? Yeah, Right!

You're probably wondering how anyone can control their weight without willpower. I know this crazy idea is exactly the opposite of what you've been told before. It's always the same deal: You want to lose ten pounds by the prom, so you promise yourself that you're going to be good. For two weeks you eat salad at every

---

Jay's Definition of Willpower

UNTITLED MESSAGE

---

willpower \ wil-pau-er \ *n.*   The first thing you lose when you go on a diet or start an exercise program. The "I'll grit my teeth and fight through this" speech that you give yourself.

➡reply to this message ➡add to favorites ➡view all replies

---

meal and trade your Twizzlers for an apple. Meanwhile, everyone else around you chows Taco Bell and Krispy Kreme donuts. But that's not a problem. All it takes to resist joining in is a little willpower, right? Hardly. Willpower doesn't work, because it doesn't last. Getting all pumped up to cut carbs and fit into your BCBG prom dress might be enough motivation for a little while, but one too many buckets of buttered popcorn sitting right there next to you in your friend's lap, smelling so good that you can't even concentrate on the movie, and you're bound to crack. Some days you have willpower, and some days you don't. It almost always fizzles out eventually. Wouldn't life be so much easier if you didn't have to rely on willpower to get the body you want?

Well, lucky for you, you don't have to. What you need to do is stop relying on willpower and start creating a permanent lifestyle where you can't help but change and stay in healthy shape.

So how do you do that?

You have to put your weight management on high priority. I call it putting yourself on "project status."

When your weight is on project status, that means you have a specific plan and you commit to it. It means you devote time and energy to the plan because it takes on special significance.

Where do you get this plan?

The plan for managing your weight is found in the seven keys.

No matter what your eating issues are, the seven keys will help you manage your weight, take better care of yourself, and do it by creating a lifestyle that supports being healthy and in shape. Even when you feel like giving up and giving in, everything in your world—how you think, how you feel, how you act—will work to keep you strong and in control.

With the seven keys, you don't need willpower because you are going to set your life up in such a way that you will be successful even when you don't necessarily *want* to do the things that will make you reach your goals.

I don't care how many diets you've been on or how many programs you've tried, with the seven keys and the steps they give you, this time you will make it. This time you will:

- Get control of your weight.

- Find exercise you actually like.

- Stop unhealthy behaviors.

- Love the body you're living in.

- Overcome food obsessions and addictions.

- Learn to love and accept yourself.

- Put more fun in your life.

As we go through this book together, I do suggest that you start a for-your-eyes-only journal where you write things down. Writing things down is a tremendous form of self-therapy because it lets you get in touch with important insights into yourself. This is an important part of putting your weight on project status.

No More Weight Worries—Freedom at Last!

Right now, you probably feel that your problems with food have you locked in your own personal prison. Trust me on this: The seven keys will unlock the door to your jail cell. You'll be free to eat things that you felt guilty about eating before. Free to enjoy your food. Free from bingeing, purging, or starving yourself. Free from the need to lie about what you ate. Free from diets. Free from obsessions with weight. Mostly, you will just be free to live a great life. Ah . . . Won't that be amazing!

Okay, okay, I know you're ready to just get to it already. But you really will have to be patient if you want to change your life. You need to take it one step at a time if you want the new you to stick.

First, we'll deal with something that's real important to managing your weight: *Your Body Image.*

Here's what's important . . .

Chapter 2

Your Body Image

want to let you in on a conversation I recently had with Amanda, a gymnast at her high school. Just so you get the picture, Amanda is 15 years old, 5 feet 3 inches, 112 pounds, and in really good shape. Sounds great to you, right? Well, Amanda thinks she's fat and is always on a diet.

Jay: How did all this start?

Amanda: I had a gymnastics coach when I was 12 who told me I was getting fat. I began hearing those words over and over in my head every time I ate. They began to really bother me. So I started skipping meals because I didn't know what else to do. Now I try different diets and pop diet pills. Sometimes I chew up my food and spit it out so I can taste it but don't have to have the calories. After school I go to gymnastics practice and make myself work out really hard, even after practice is over. I can't concentrate on much else but losing weight.

Jay: So this is how you try to control your weight?

Amanda: Yes.

Jay: If you're always on a diet, how are your energy level and performance for gymnastics?

Amanda: Not that great. Sometimes I feel so weak that I think it will be a miracle if I make it through practice without collapsing. I've got a lot of pain in my legs. It scares me because if I have to drop out of gymnastics, I'll probably get fatter and fatter. So I work through the pain and try to ignore it.

Jay: You really think you're fat?

Amanda: Yes, compared to my friends. I constantly compare myself to other girls at school, too, girls who are drop-dead gorgeous. Or I go to the mall and look at other girls' bodies and say in my mind, "She's fatter than me . . . she's skinnier than me." I'm not anywhere near thin. I've always felt that I need to weigh 100 pounds. When I look in the mirror, I see someone who needs to lose weight. I cry and beat myself up over it and think I look so bad. I want to be skinnier with a flatter stomach and smaller hips. There are bunch of things I want to change about my body.

Jay: So you weigh about 112 now? And you feel fat?

Amanda: I would love to be thinner. Then I'd be prettier and more popular. I just see myself as fat, and fat is terrible.

Jay: Do you realize that you don't look fat? Have people said you're not fat?

Amanda: Yes. But they're just being nice. I'm sure they see me the way I see myself—fat. I just want to be thinner, and that's all I care about.

Maybe you can relate to what Amanda is saying. Do you think you're fat even though you're at a totally normal weight? Are you trying to diet down to an unrealistic weight? Do you hate what you see in the mirror?

Like so many teens today—and maybe like you—Amanda is thin but sees herself as fat. She wants to get to what is an unrealistic and possibly unhealthy weight because she can't accept her own body. Amanda has a "body image" problem.

What Is Body Image, Anyway?

My psychological team set me straight on this one: Body image has to do with how you see your body in your mind's eye. It also has to with how you talk to yourself and others about your body, how you feel about your body, and how you treat it. In short, it's an inside view of your outside self.

Body image can be positive or negative. If you have a poor body image, you might think you're too fat, too skinny, not pretty enough, or not muscular enough. Having a negative body image means not accepting your body the way it is, focusing on what you think are your flaws, and putting yourself down because of them.

When you get hung up on your body's imperfections—which everyone has because no body is perfect—you may start sabotaging yourself in all kinds of unhealthy ways. For example:

- Not eating.

- Going on crash diets that don't work, and never will.

- Obsessing over everything you eat and feeling guilty about it.

- Worrying about your appearance, rather than enjoying your life.

If your body image is positive, that means you like and accept your body the way it is. With a positive body image, you require more of yourself, respecting and taking care of your body. So you eat good foods. You exercise or play sports because they make you feel good. You don't spend your life obsessing over the 3.2 pounds you gained last month. If you have a good body image, you'll feel more confident that you can get in shape. This is a healthy attitude that gives you a lot of power to start taking real control over your weight.

Body Image and Self-Image—What's the Difference?

A lot of people confuse body image with self-image. Self-image has to do with how you see all of you—your personality, strengths, talents, interests, skills, abilities, attitudes, and other personal qualities. That "view of you" can be true—meaning that you're truly happy and at peace with yourself. Or it can be really screwed up, because you've let people and experiences make you doubt yourself, your worth, and your value. You might feel inferior in a lot of ways because you started believing negative comments made about you. Or you compare yourself to other people, never quite measuring up to what you think is the mark. All of these things can shape a poor self-image. A poor self-image can fill you up with a lot of negative feelings.

Having a good self-image, on the other hand, is important because when you believe in yourself, you're less likely to let your own mistakes, or criticisms from other people, get you down. You don't compare yourself to other people. With a good self-image, it's easier to go after and achieve your goals. You see yourself as a winner, so you act like a winner. You treat yourself with dignity and respect. You have the conviction that you're special and unique, and believing this in your heart and mind gives you the chance to live a really great life.

So where does body image fit in? Body image is just one part of your self-image, but it's a pretty key part because it does affect how you view yourself. When you feel attractive, you act more confident. People start sizing you up more positively because that's how you present yourself to the world. Feeling good about your body and your appearance can help you feel good about yourself.

What's Your Body Image?

What about you? How much of what you see in the mirror do you like or dislike? How does your body image shape up?

Let's begin to find out here with a short ten-question quiz. Answer each question with yes or no. Be honest, even if it hurts.

1. Do you avoid mirrors when walking by them?
2. Do you hate wearing a bathing suit at the pool, beach, or some other public place?
3. Do you wear clothes that will hide or disguise parts of your body?
4. Do you dislike having your picture taken?
5. Have you ever postponed shopping for new clothes until you've lost weight?
6. Do you feel ashamed of your body a lot of the time?
7. Do you think your breasts are (too big) (too small) (some other putdown)?
8. When you're hanging out with a friend who you think has a better body than yours, do you feel bad?

9. Do you often compare your body to the bodies of models and celebrities in the media?

10. Do you usually ignore compliments from other people about your appearance?

Scoring

Count up the number of times you answered yes and the number of times you answered no. If you have only 0 to 2 yeses, and the rest noes, you have a positive body image. That's a plus, because when you accept and appreciate your body, you treat it that way.

If you have more than two yeses, your body image may be negative. You may feel uncomfortable with your body, and you may worry too much about what you look like. Not liking your body only sets you up for unhappiness, stress, and weight problems.

Body image is a big deal. It's something you can change. You can learn to love your body so much that you'll want to take care of it—and that's what we'll work on here, and throughout all the keys.

How to Feel Better About Your Body

Most teens do want to feel better about themselves. In the survey I conducted, I found that a lot of teens think they have to change how they look in order to feel good about themselves. But that's not it. Changing your attitude toward your body—not changing your body—is one of the secrets toward feeling good about yourself. When you feel good about yourself, you can do what it takes to require more of yourself in terms of your weight and health.

How can you go about doing that? How can you avoid feeling so bad about how you look? How can you change your body image?

What's important to do first is realize that your body image is influenced by a lot of different forces in your life. Here are some of them:

- The media, which projects images of bodies that are unrealistically thin and may lead you to believe there is something wrong with you because you don't look like the super-thin supermodels.

- Negative, hurtful teasing from your peers or family, which can harm your body image and make you feel bad about your appearance.

- Parents who think negatively about their own bodies and therefore set a bad example for you.

- Your own inner dialogue—the way you talk to yourself about your body.

Once you see that these things are working against you, you've got to do something about them. Here's how.

Step 1: Get Real About the Media

You and I and everybody else live in a Hollywood-ized world where the "ideal body" is plastered all over our TVs, the movies, magazines, and billboards. Images of the perfect babes and hunks are pressuring us to be thin and good-looking. Yet every one of these images ignores the fact that we come in a wide assortment of pleasing sizes and shapes.

Do something for me right now. Go get one of your magazines. Check out the girls on the cover. I bet you think they look pretty great, right?

Well, I've got some news for you. I've worked with these magazines and I do TV shows. What you see in the media isn't real. Photographs are retouched to the point where complexions can be cleared up. Thighs can be slimmed down. Hair can be added. TV cameras even have beauty lenses that take away flaws!

These unreal media images can create real problems for you at this time in your life. The medical doctors I worked with on this book explained this to me: If you're a girl, you started a growth spurt around 12 or 13, and you'll keep on spurting right on through to 15 or 16. By the time you're physically mature, you'll add roughly 25 percent body fat to your figure. Some of it goes to your breasts, but a lot of it heads straight to your hips and thighs. I know that's probably not what you want to hear, but that fat is part of your natural development.

Unfortunately, it's right around the time your body is changing and filling out that you start reading magazines and seeing movies and TV shows with those "skinny equals beautiful" messages. You know what? You're being bombarded with these messages at a time when your body is not developing that way! So you're entering a world where, by media standards, you look less than perfect. But it's total bull. What the media is telling you is normal is *not* normal.

Guys, you're a target too. The same messages making your girlfriend feel like she needs to be thinner are brainwashing you into thinking you need six-pack abs and serious pecs to be good-looking. Unfortunately a lot of guys are willing to do it at any cost, including using steroids and compulsively spending endless hours in the gym. And no matter how big your muscles get, maybe you start thinking it's still not big enough.

It's so easy to buy into the belief that your body needs to look a certain way in order for you to feel good about yourself. Think about all those ads you see. They all star really cute girls and guys with great skin and perfect bodies, laughing like their lives are all friends and fun all the time. Eventually you start to wonder why your life doesn't look like that. You think, maybe if I could wear the same Low Rise Levi's and have that same flat stomach, I'd be happy and popular too. And that's exactly what the advertisers want—they rely on you wanting to be just like the models and stars who use or wear their products.

What this all means is that when you are comparing yourself to media images, you are comparing yourself to a fantasy. You are going to lose that contest 100 out of 100 times. Comparing yourself to what you see in the media can have a very negative effect on your body image. Maybe you might want to stop buying fashion magazines, at least for the time that you are working on your body image and can view this stuff for what it is—totally unreal!

Focus on who you are on the inside, not on your outward appearance. Your body is only one part of you. You have so many other things to offer!

Don't get me wrong, it is okay and actually good for you to want to look good, dress well, and have a nice appearance. I'm not saying we shouldn't try to look good. We should. I work out and try to dress well just like everybody else, but I also eat ice cream and I don't live in the gym. There is nothing wrong with wanting to look good, but we need to have goals other than looking like Courteney Cox from *Friends*.

Step 2: Stand Up Against Teasing

Teasing by peers and families over weight is devastating to body image—and to lives. In fact, suicide and other emotional problems like depression disturb teens who are teased about their weight, according to some really serious research I looked into on this subject. The study I read says that kids who get teased about their weight are two to three times more likely to consider suicide, or actually follow through on it.

Teasing is a sick and nasty game. The really destructive thing about teasing is when you hear time and time again that you're a fat butterball or a big ass, it becomes part of your nature, and it lives on in your mind. It causes you to hate your body. It can diminish your confidence and make you feel angry and bitter. It makes you feel so shut out and rejected that you feel like you can't do or say anything.

But you can. As we go through the seven keys together, you're going to learn to un-internalize this stuff, move it aside, and become the person you really are. That's a preview of coming attractions, but what about right now?

When someone teases you, calling you rude and hurtful names, the first thing to remember is that their comment says nothing about you, only about them. People who feel bad about themselves try to make up for their own insecurities and self-doubt by putting other people down. Please get this so you can see through their bull and not believe what they say.

If you're getting teased, you've got to be ready with some comebacks. Standing up for yourself in a calm, confident, and nonsarcastic way will help you get control and feel better about yourself. It will help prevent your body image and your psyche from getting further damaged. Some good comebacks to teasing are to:

- Respond with a compliment, acting like the comment is made out of genuine concern for you. Example:

Teaser: If you eat that, you'll get fat.

You: That's really nice of you to let me know. It's cool that you care so much about me.

- Agree with part of the remark. We all know the whole truth about ourselves, good or bad. We know our weak points and our flaws, so if there's an ounce of truth in the teasing, agree with that bit of truth. Admitting a weakness knocks the wind out of a teaser's sails. Example:

Teaser: You eat like a pig.

You: Yeah, you're right, I do eat a lot.

- Respond with humor. A humorous comeback is always a great defense—practically guaranteed to take the bite out of teasing. Example:

Teaser: A picture of you would weigh ten pounds.

You: That's so old. I fell off my dinosaur when I first heard it.

- Say thanks. Treat the comment with appreciation—like the teaser is doing you a favor. Example:

Teaser: You look like you've gained weight.

You: Thanks! I'm glad you noticed.

It's a good idea to plan and practice your responses, maybe working with someone you trust. Let's give this a try. How would you respond to the following? Write your answer in the spaces provided.

You'd be so much prettier if you lost a little weight.

_____

_____

_____

You've had enough for dinner. You'll get fat.

_____

_____

_____

There just isn't anywhere for all of that food to go, you better watch it.

_____

_____

_____

Hey, wide load!

_____

_____

_____

You'll learn more skills for dealing with these situations as we go through this book. But there is one more action you can take, and we'll talk more about it Key 2. That action is forgiveness.

When someone teases you in a hurtful way, it is only natural that you have a negative reaction like anger, humiliation, or bitterness. Such emotions are so powerful that when they are present, they change who you are and push all other feelings and emotions to the background. An ugly comment hurts—and hurts for a long time afterward. The hurt not only causes an ouch, but there is a re-ouch every time you think about it.

One of the best things you can do is let the hurt, the anger, or the bitterness go. You can do this by forgiving. Does this mean that I'm telling you to go to the person who has hurt you and say, "I forgive you"? No way. The forgiveness I'm talking about is all about you and not about whoever has hurt you. These people don't even have to know that you've forgiven them. This forgiveness is something that takes place within you and for you. By forgiving the people who have hurt you, you free yourself. If you let what they said to you ruin your life, then they've won. Don't let that happen.

Step 3: Recognize Your Parents' Influence on Your Body Image

Sometimes parents don't help either. When your mom stands in front of the mirror and says, "These pants make me look so fat," what do you think that is teaching you? It's teaching you that demeaning your body, treating it with less respect, is okay.

Casey is the perfect example of this. She grew up in a house and with a mom who constantly taught her to hate her body. I recently sat down with her and she told me all about what it is like to live in that type of a house. Look at some of what she had to say:

Viewing Options: ➡view all messages ➡view all messages ➡outline view

UNTITLED MESSAGE

Mom was always on or off a diet, so I was raised that thinness is a way of life—something to strive for, always. I guess I just learned to *always* examine myself because it seemed that that is what my mom did. She always asked us if her butt looked big and then insisted that it did. No matter how skinny she gets she still "hates" her body. She even tells me, "Casey, you better hope that you didn't get my hips!" She talks about how she has fasted for days, gone on all-liquid diets, eaten nothing but fruit, all of this crazy stuff and none of it has worked.

After all of this I am terrified of gaining weight. Plus, I feel that if I want to be "one of the girls," I too have to hate my body.

And then my mom keeps telling me that I better catch it early and figure something out before I look like her because once I do it will never change. So I kept going on diets, too, but I hated it. I rebelled and started bingeing mindlessly on chips, ice cream, cookies—whatever I could sneak into the house. I've gained, like, forty pounds in the past two years. I feel so weak for not being able to control myself and stay on a diet. But I do not want to gain any more weight. I want to lose weight, but I have no idea what to do. My mom has taught me how to hate the body I have, but she never did teach me any-thing about how to have a body I love.

➡reply to this message ➡add to favorites ➡view all replies

Recognize if your parents have maybe been not-so-hot role models, but realize that you can't change them. The best move you can make here is to work on changing yourself and hope that your efforts will inspire a positive response from the other side. If it does, all the better. If you're trying to work on things like body image or your weight, it helps if you've got support from your parents. When a parent offers either to join in the plan or to do something similar, this is a very powerful win-win sort of bonding. (You'll learn more on parental support-building in Key 7.)

Step 4: Stop Body Bashing

No one likes a braggart. I knew a guy in high school who used to brag about everything: his car, his clothes, his afterschool job, etc. If BS was music, he could have been the whole school band. He obviously did this to try to impress us, when in fact we'd just roll our eyes after he left.

The one time when it's okay—and a good thing, really—to brag is to yourself about yourself. We just don't do it enough. If we did, our body images wouldn't be so screwed up.

You can start changing your body image by starting to brag about yourself and your appearance more often, to yourself. Remember my saying that your body image is formed by your attitudes and feelings toward your body? That's really good news because you can change your body image by challenging and changing those attitudes. We'll talk more about this in Key 1—how to change your negative self-talk—because it's really central to everything we'll be doing in this book. If you're always criticizing your body, think of the devastating effect this can have. When you're ready to improve your diet or start an exercise program, and all of your thoughts are saying things like "I'm too fat to be seen at the gym," and "I always look terrible," and "I'm disgusted with my body," you'll avoid situations and taking action because of the way you feel about your body.

So you've got to stop saying negative things about your body and start giving yourself compliments. For example:

"I appreciate the beauty of my own body."

"I don't need to be thin to look good."

"My body is unique and special."

"My body is strong. It lets me walk, run, play, and dance."

In the space below or in your journal, list what you like about your body and your appearance.

_____

_____

When you start to have a bad attitude about your body, read what you wrote about yourself. This and the other steps you've learned here will help you treat yourself as the treasure you are.

You Gotta Get Real About Your Body

Working on your body image is an ongoing project. It doesn't change overnight. Changes come slowly, but they come. And when they do, you'll feel so much better about your body, in a way you never knew you could feel. And remember, the better your body image, the better you'll take care of yourself and treat yourself.

Before moving on, I want you to meet a couple of teens who got real about their bodies and got their lives together:

Viewing Options: ➡ view all messages ➡ view all messages ➡ outline view

UNTITLED MESSAGE

I started gaining weight in the tenth grade, and my boobs were getting big too. I wore baggy clothes to hide my body. I couldn't stand to look at myself in the mirror. Right around the time I was thinking about going on a diet, my older brother asked me if I wanted to go to the gym with him and try lifting weights. At first I didn't want to because I had tried lots of different exercise stuff before, but nothing seemed to work. But I agreed to give it a try, and I liked it that I could wear baggy sweatclothes. After about three weeks of working out with my brother, something pretty crazy happened. Biceps appeared in my arms. I didn't know I had muscles, and I sure didn't know they could develop that fast. I was totally hooked. When the rest of me began to get toned up in a matter of weeks, I started valuing my body because of its strength and beauty. I don't feel self-conscious anymore, and I've traded my baggy sweatshirt for just a sports bra. I never did have to go on that diet. I can finally look in the mirror and like what I see. Trying to be "perfect" is a waste of what little time I have to spend on myself. There's no such thing as a perfect body. You have to do what's best for your health and well-being. If I can feel like this, anyone can.
—Suze, age 16

Sure, I wish I weighed a little less. Heck, I can gain weight just driving by a store that sells Twinkies. But so what? I know I'll never be on the cover of a magazine. I don't fixate on my faults. Instead, I try to describe myself in ways that have nothing to do with my body or how I look. Adjectives like caring, giving, loving, intelligent, compassionate, a good sport, loyal to my friends come to mind. When you get right down to it, it's better to be complimented on your personality than on your clothes. You don't need to be anything or anyone different than who you are.

—James, age 17

➡reply to this message ➡add to favorites ➡view all replies

Like these teens, you have to get honest with yourself about your body and what you can really look like. Maximize the best of you. Do the best you can with everything you have. Trust me, once you do this, you'll start feeling good about yourself and about your life. You'll start looking good and feeling better because you're treating yourself the way you deserve to be treated, without being obsessed with what you eat or how you look.

There are great changes ahead of you. Now you just need some realistic goals for getting there. What you really want is within reach. Goals give you the power to get it.

Chapter 3

Get-With-It Goals

hen I was in high school, I knew that I wanted to go to law school one day. I was familiar with the legal profession because my dad was involved in the strategic planning of legal cases, and I absolutely loved it. Sometimes all I could think about was the day when I would get to go. But there was something standing between me and my law school career: college. If it were up to me, I would have skipped undergraduate school altogether. But life and academics don't work like that (unless you're lucky enough to be an Einstein who can finish college in the time it takes most of us to find our way around the dorm).

My focus—going to law school—ultimately led me to map out my college career, so that I could finish in three years, rather than the usual four or five. This plan meant taking certain steps each year: carrying a super-heavy course load every semester, going to summer school, working a million assignments, and cramming like heck for tests. A lot of the time, I absolutely hated it and wanted to quit. But as hard as it was, I did it to accomplish my ultimate goal of getting to law school as soon as possible. I didn't always work efficiently toward that goal; sometimes I slacked off by not studying as hard as I could have but instead going out with my friends. But I always got myself back on track because I knew what I wanted, and I knew what it would take to get it.

My goal was to get to law school. What about you? Do you know what you want? Do you know where you're going or what you're working toward?

Most people don't know how to answer these questions because they don't have a clue what it is they really want. They don't know anything about setting goals, or taking steps to achieve them. Well, now it's time to fix that.

What Is the Big Deal About Goals?

A goal is something you really desire, something you're willing to work for. Maybe you want to make the cheerleading team or varsity football. Maybe you want a new car. Maybe you want to go to college. Maybe you want to be healthier. There are as many goals out there as there are people who set them. The important thing about goals is that they be meaningful for you.

Setting goals isn't just another thing for you to do. It's what you do to get something more out of life. If you think setting goals sounds boring and is barely worth a yawn, it's time for a wakeup call: Being successful isn't boring, and if you want to be successful, you need to spend time on goal setting. If you're not totally convinced, check out the box "Why Goals Matter" on page 36 for a little convincing.

The need to set goals is relevant to everything you do. If you want to create your ideal life; if you want to succeed in anything, then you have to have goals to get you there. Although the goals we'll be defining in this chapter focus on your weight, fitness, and health, what you'll learn applies to anything and everything you want out of life. So listen carefully!

Goals Are What Make Your Dreams Come True

We all dream about what might be. We all fantasize about what we want to look like, where we want to go, how we want to live. It's

Why Goals Matter

- Goals give your life meaning and purpose.
- Goals help you develop control over your own destiny.
- Goals help you get more of what you want and less of what you don't want.
- Goals bump you out of your comfort zone and help you reach for more.
- Goals help you fight peer pressure because you're working toward what you want, not what others want.
- Goals, and making them, increase your chances of success.
- Goals help you recognize which choices support what you want and which do not.
- Goals provide a game plan for making your dreams come true.
- Goals teach you to believe in yourself and give you confidence.
- Goals give you the power to create your own future.

fun to let our imaginations run wild. But how about turning these dreams into reality?

You do that by turning those dreams into goals. The big difference between a dream and a goal is that dreams are kind of fuzzy and vague, and goals are very clear and specific. Dreams are all about something you long for. Goals involve a strategic plan for getting there.

Wishing you could lose ten pounds doesn't make you look better in a bathing suit. Fantasizing that you made the team doesn't get you in shape for the season. Dreaming about what you want in the future doesn't get you there, goal setting does. When your life is defined in relation to your goals, you're focused and energized. You just have to know how to turn your dreams into goals. Here's how.

Step 1: Translate Your Dream Into Specific Events or Behaviors That Define What You Want

It is not enough to say that you want to be in better shape. You have to define "better shape" specifically or behaviorally. What does it mean in the real world? What will you be doing or not doing when you are living the goal? How will you recognize it when you have it?

What you have to do is create a *goal statement* for yourself. For example:

> *"I intend to get more toned or more muscular such that I can* **bench-press 185 pounds** *and* **run an eight-minute mile** *by* **joining a gym** *and* **working out with weights three times a week for six weeks,** *and I will create rewards for my compliance so that I don't quit when I start to lose my motivation."*

When your dream has been broken down into behaviors, or actions, those specific goals are much easier to manage and pursue than a dream world statement like "I want to get in better shape."

One warning: There are going to be big temptations and peer pressure for you to stick to your old ways. So your goals have to include specifics about how to keep yourself out of situations where the pressure is going to be intense. When creating a goal statement for yourself, leave no room for confusion about what you want.

So, in your goal statement you need to include:

- **Exactly and specifically what you want.**

- **How you plan to get it.**

- **When it will happen.**

- **What you will do to prevent failure.**

If you think through your goal and you write it down as a goal statement, then I promise that your chances of success increase greatly.

Step 2: Translate Your Dream Into Things You Can Measure

A goal needs to be measurable; that is, you've got to be able to quantify it by attaching a realistic number to it. In the dream world, you might say, "I want to fit into my jeans again." In the world of goals, you need to define "fitting into your jeans" the same way I defined "more toned or more muscular" in Step 1, in terms that are measurable. What size are those jeans? What measurements do you want to have? How many pounds must you lose? Translate your dream into what you can measure.

This dimension of goal setting helps you monitor the progress you're making toward your goal. Day by day, week by week, month by month, you can see how much of the goal you've attained, how close you are or how far you still have to go, and whether you've met your goal or not. When your goal is measurable, you'll know exactly when you've reached it—then you can get psyched, tell your friends, pat yourself on the back, and celebrate! Just as you saw in Step 1, your definition of success has to be specific and measurable. Remember however, that the definition can be behavioral (I will work out three times a week) or results-oriented (the ability to run an eight-minute mile). But whatever the goal is, it must be specific and measurable.

Step 3: Assign a Time Line to Your Goal

Unlike dreams, which are fuzzy in both definition and time, goals require a schedule. Using my Step 1 example again, a dream world statement is "I want to get in better shape." A goal statement sounds like "I want to lose 15 pounds by June 1" or "I want to be able to do 65 push-ups by basketball season."

Be sure to create a *reasonable* time frame to reach your goal. Trying to lose 15 pounds in two weeks is practically impossible—and totally unhealthy. You really need about eight weeks. If your goal is to lose 15 pounds by June 1, your start date should be April 5 or earlier. Working from that date, you can see where you have to be at the midpoint four-week mark. Thinking in terms of a calendar lets you see what you need to keep doing each day to reach your goal. While you have to be reasonable in giving yourself enough time to lose the weight, you also have to be reasonable in that you don't give yourself too much time. If you give yourself an entire year to lose 7 pounds, then the benefit of a time line is lost. So, be reasonable on both ends of the continuum.

A schedule of achievement, marked on a calendar or in a daily planner, will keep you motivated. You have to make a commitment to what you want and when. By setting a time line to your goal, you will hold yourself to a schedule rather than just wishing it will happen. This step is *very* important.

Step 4: Choose a Goal That You Can Control

Unlike dreams, in which you fantasize about all different things, some of which you can't possibly control, like winning the lottery or taking Justin Timberlake to the prom, a goal has to involve things to which you have access and therefore can manipulate. If what you want is to look tall and lean like Cameron Diaz and your natural body type is short and curvy, chances are you need to set a different goal. You have no control over the outcome—you can't change your height, and you can't healthfully get super-lean because your DNA has programmed you to have hips and a butt. Cameron is just not an appropriate or realistic goal for you. However, what you can do is control what you eat, how often you exercise, how you treat your body, or what you wear to look as attractive as you can. If you want to look like a Charlie's Angel, maybe you'll have to aim for more of a Drew Barrymore bod. You can control things that maximize what you have.

When you set your goal around what you control, your chances of achieving it go way up. If your success depends solely on the actions of others, then that is a bad goal. I once made the goal that I was going to get my aunt to quit smoking. I knew that smoking was really stupid and that it would kill her, but the decision to give up smoking was totally out of my control and I failed because she made the decision not to quit. Now a reasonable goal could have been to make a deal with myself that she wouldn't smoke in the same room as me. I control the success of this goal because I have the ability to leave the room if she insists on smoking. Because I control my success on this goal it is a good goal to have made. So, when you are picking your goals, make sure that your success is not totally within the control of someone else.

Step 5: Plan a Program and a Strategy That Will Get You to Your Goal

If you don't have a plan to get you from where you are to where you want to be, you will never get there. Think of what would happen if you tried to get to an address in another state without directions or a map. You'd get so lost that you'd have to run an ad in the paper for someone to come and find you. But if you had a map, with clear directions and landmarks, you'd get there. Have a strategy to reach your goals, and you will get where you want to go.

Plus, when you have a strategy in place, you don't have to depend on willpower. Willpower doesn't work anyway, because it fizzles out, and you're back to where you started.

So what would a goal-oriented strategy look like? It might require:

- Eating out at a fast-food restaurant once a week, instead of three—or ten.

- Negotiating with your parents so they buy healthier foods.

- Stopping your self-critical thinking by saying positive, respectful things and affirming what you like about your body.

- Learning how to handle stress productively, without turning to food.

- Setting aside a specific time of the day to exercise, and not letting anything else get in the way during that period.

With a strategy in place, your weight is on project status to carry you through when willpower fades away. With every key in this book, you'll learn how to do that. The strategy for achieving the goal in Step 1 was working out three times a week. A strategy for making better grades might be to study at least two hours each school day. Whatever your goal, set an action plan such that you can strategically pursue your goal.

Step 6: Define Your Goal in Terms of Steps

A really effective goal-setting strategy involves breaking your goal into manageable steps that lead to what you ultimately want. Achieving that goal will be the product of lots of small steps made each day. It won't be some giant leap you make all at once—that's way too overwhelming. Losing 100 pounds may seem impossible, but losing 10 pounds in six weeks probably doesn't. So, instead of trying to lose 100 pounds, maybe you should look at your goal as losing 10 pounds, ten times. This most likely seems much more doable. These small steps represent your short-term goals. Short-term goals are smaller goals you can reach in a day, a week, or a month. They keep you moving toward your bigger goal, sometimes called a "long-term goal."

I can't tell you in this book what your little steps should be; only you can do that. But I can give you some pretty clear examples to point you in the right direction. Let's say you don't want to be overweight anymore. You want to feel proud of your body. That's a great goal. But sometimes our big goals feel so overwhelming they can be paralyzing. Big goals, though, begin to look much more doable when broken down into smaller steps. So figure out what your steps will be before you set out. These steps could be:

- Eating a fresh fruit at lunch.

- Having two servings of fresh vegetables every day.

- Switching to Diet Coke instead of regular Coke.

- Losing a pound a week.

- Cutting back on your TV time and doing something active instead.

So work toward your goal in small steps, not huge leaps. Each positive step you take can be counted as a success—and each one will feel better than the last!

Step 7: Create Accountability Toward the Progress of Your Goal

Figure out some way to hold yourself accountable for what you say you are going to do. Maybe you tell a friend about your plan and have her ask how it's going once a week. Or maybe you require yourself to write down your progress every day in your journal. So you can monitor where you are, maybe you put a daily progress and accountability chart on the refrigerator. Whatever way, make sure that you have to be made accountable on a regular basis.

Support from someone you trust helps you reach your goals too. That support can take various forms. It can be arranging a ride to exercise class; getting money from your parents for a gym membership; taking advice from a trainer, coach, or mentor; or receiving encouragement from a friend to keep you going on those days when you don't feel like working on your goal. Setting up a system of accountability for yourself makes it impossible for you *not* to reach your goal.

Now It's Your Turn

Let's make our discussion of goal setting personal and practical. In your journal or in the space below, write out your goals according to the seven steps outlined above. Feel free to add to this plan as you learn and use the seven keys.

Step 1: Translate your dream into specific events or behaviors. Specifically what is it you want to achieve? What are the specific behaviors or actions that make up this goal? How will you recognize it when you get there? What will you do to prevent failure? What is your goal date?

_____

_____

_____

_____

_____

Step 2: Translate your dream into things that you can measure, such as how many pounds you want to lose and what weight you'd like to achieve. Again, make sure this weight is realistic for your height and body type. Or, if your goal is to exercise regularly, make sure you write down exactly how many days a week you will exercise, how many miles you'll run every day, or how many sets of sit-ups you'll do. Whatever the goal or goals, make sure you can measure your progress and your success.

_____

_____

_____

_____

Step 3: Assign a time line for achieving your goal, and write it in the space below. Transfer this information to your calendar or daily planner. Include both your short-term and your long-term, or ultimate, goals.

Goals:

Dates:

Step 4: Choose a goal you can control. Review what you have written so far. To check if your goal is something you can control, ask yourself: Do I feel I can achieve this? Is it realistic for me? Are the circumstances within my control? If not, reword your goal so that it reflects things you can control.

_____

_____

_____

_____

_____

Step 5: Plan a program and a strategy that will get you to your goal. What are some ways you can rearrange your life to reach your goal? Schedule exercise into your week? Finding new things to do so you'll be less preoccupied with food, dieting, and weight? Identifying ways to avoid temptations and peer pressure for you to stick to your old ways? (As we go through this book together, you'll find some excellent strategies to add to this list!)

_____

_____

_____

_____

_____

Step 6: Define your goal in terms of steps. Remember, you've got to accomplish a series of smaller goals, one by one, in order to reach the big one. What small steps will you take to reach your goal? Write them down in the space below.

_____

_____

_____

_____

_____

Step 7: Be accountable for your progress toward your goal. In the space below, list some people in your life who might be helpful for support and keeping you accountable. Also list any other methods you plan to use like marking your calendar "yes" or "no" every day to indicate whether or not you worked toward your goal that day.

_____

_____

_____

_____

_____

Special Bulletin: If You've Got an Eating Disorder

When I was researching this book and writing this chapter, my psychological consultants advised me to be very clear, careful, and specific about goal setting for anyone who may be in the grip of an eating disorder like anorexia or bulimia. In these cases, setting *appropriate* goals for getting well is not just important, it can be life-saving.

So read the following with both eyes and with your full attention. If you suffer from bulimia, don't set a goal to lose weight by using extreme measures like throwing up or taking laxatives. Better goals would be to stop bingeing, vomiting, or using laxatives, or to use food as good nutrition, to take care of your body.

If you're suffering from anorexia, a vital goal might be to gain weight, maybe as little as one pound a week. This is also something you need to work on with the help of a therapist, a doctor, and your parents. As with someone who has bulimia, stopping behaviors like starving or purging are appropriate, and indeed necessary, goals if you have anorexia.

Another healthy and appropriate goal for someone with an eating disorder is to *restore healthy eating*. What does that goal look like? Maybe it means you eat three healthy and enjoyable meals each day. Maybe it means you get your focus off food and weight and have fun doing other things. Maybe it means that you eat when you're hungry and stop eating when you're full. Maybe it means going to McDonald's a couple of times and not feeling guilty about it. Whatever the eating disorder, the ultimate goal is getting well, and there are many small, short-term goals you can set to get there. Follow the same seven steps for reaching this goal and also ask a professional for help and advice.

Feel Good About Yourself

Pursuing the wrong goals can be a big mistake. Many teens, especially girls, fixate on dieting and getting thin, wanting to look like supermodels. They think that if they look like supermodels, they'll feel better about themselves.

Misstating your goals can be an incredibly devastating problem if you can't have the look you want. Here's an example of what I'm talking about: If you decide the only thing that can make you happy is to look like Jennifer Aniston or Brad Pitt, chances are that's not going to happen. If you remain overly focused on that desire, you can spend your whole life being frustrated, because you may never achieve that goal. It may not be possible. And that frustration might make you do some really dumb things, like criticizing your body all the time or going on some extreme and dangerous diet.

But what did you really want in this instance? The truth is that you probably want to have the feelings that come from looking like Jen or Brad. What you really want is to feel attractive, handsome, confident, beautiful, or proud of your body.

But here's the deal: It's important to go for the feelings, not the ridiculously thin thighs that you think will give you the feelings. By refusing to become fixated on looking like someone else, you give yourself a lot more flexibility for getting what you want. If you are smart enough to realize that you want the feelings you think will come from looking like a celebrity, then you can find any number of more realistic and healthier ways to get those feelings. There may be hundreds of ways to get those feelings that have nothing to do with trying to look like someone else. You could start treating your body with love and respect. You could change your hairstyle. You could get some new clothes. You could start an exercise program to get more in touch with your physical self. You could start changing your self-critical nature by practicing true, positive thinking. There are plenty of things you can do to make yourself feel like a star without changing your body.

I've talked to a lot of teens who are obsessed with seeing a certain number when they step on the scale. Melinda, 18, was a really good example. Like so many other girls, she had locked in on a target weight—102 pounds—as what she wanted to achieve rather than focusing on feelings and experiences. In talking to Melinda, I wanted her to realize that what she wanted was not some magic number like 102, which was probably too thin for her anyway. Instead what she wanted was the feeling she decided weighing 102 pounds would bring her. Here's a brief clip from our conversation.

Jay: Melinda, what is it you're shooting for?

Melinda: I want to weigh 102. That's my goal. I think I'll look really good at that weight.

Jay: What are you going to have to do to reach that goal?

Melinda: I'm going to have to stay on a really strict diet and exercise for a couple of hours every day.

Jay: Let's fast-forward to when you weigh 102. How will it make you feel? How will it feel to walk around at 102 pounds?

Melinda: It will feel great. I'll feel graceful, and beautiful. I'll feel really good about myself. I'll feel proud of myself.

Jay: So what you really want is to feel graceful, beautiful, and proud—basically to just feel good about yourself?

Melinda: Yeah. That's right.

Jay: Melinda, do you think there might be other ways to feel graceful, proud of yourself, and beautiful—without all the dieting and exercising? Are those the smartest choices you can make to get those feelings?

Melinda: Well, what do you mean?

Jay: Have you ever volunteered for something—you know, doing something to help somebody else?

Melinda: Sure, I volunteered at the hospital, reading to sick kids.

Jay: How did that make you feel?

Melinda: Good about myself, really good. I felt proud of myself for making other people feel good.

Jay: Have you ever treated yourself to a new haircut, new outfit or a makeover? Or have you ever exercised just for the fun of it? Do you have any special talents, like writing, painting, or playing music?

Melinda: Yeah . . . I do a lot of those things. I like changing my hair. Sometimes my friends and I play volleyball at the beach. That's fun and I'm good at it. I can play the piano too.

Jay: And you feel pretty when you change your hairstyle, right? Or confident when you work on your interests and hobbies? Proud of yourself when you volunteer? Isn't that right?

Melinda: Yes.

Jay: So feeling pretty, feeling graceful, feeling proud of your-self, feeling good about yourself doesn't have to do with a number on a scale, does it?

Melinda: No, I guess not. There are a lot of things you can do to feel good about yourself.

Melinda got it: She realized that she could get the feelings she wanted, right now, without waiting until she weighed 102 pounds. Weighing 102 pounds wasn't the road to the feelings she wanted; it was a detour. I hope you get it too. *You can feel proud of your body without weighing a certain number on the scale.* So, instead of trying to get to a certain weight, work to get the feelings that you think that weight will bring you. If you go for the feelings, your chances of success are a lot better and so too are your chances of happi-ness. The fact is, if you pick the goal of weighing 102 pounds out of the air, you may be very disappointed even if you manage to reach that goal. Weighing 102 pounds will not make you feel pretty and proud, but a lot of other things very likely will. So, look for and pur-sue the things that truly can.

Here's your chance to double-check your goals to make sure you're going after what you truly want. The pattern of questions I used in talking to Melinda goes like this:

What do you want?

What must you do to have it?

What will it feel like when you have it?

What are all the ways you can get those feelings—no mat-ter how much you weigh?

When you are answering these questions, be honest, be sincere, but most of all, be precise. When I say precise, I mean you should come up with as many different ways to arrive at those feelings as you can. The clearer you are about what you want, how you want to feel, and how to get there, the easier it will be for you to recognize whether you are taking a step in the wrong direction. If you don't know exactly what it is that you want, you will never even know if you get there. You have to be very specific about what you want, and when you are successful, don't be afraid to stand up and claim your victory.

Don't misunderstand me: There's nothing wrong with setting a goal to be a certain weight—as long as that goal is healthy and realistic for you. But make sure you can describe how you want to feel too. When you do that, you begin to see all the ways to get those feelings—things you can do, even today, without putting yourself through the torture of dieting and overexercising, or putting your life on hold until you reach some random number on a scale.

When you focus your attention on these things, you *will* start feeling good about yourself. Other people will notice that—in the way you carry and present yourself. You'll come across with beauty and confidence because you feel good from the inside out. You don't have to change your body, or lose even a single pound, to feel better about yourself.

As you work on setting goals for yourself, be bold enough to reach for what will truly fulfill you, without being unrealistic or focusing on the wrong things. Don't be shy about saying that you want something great for yourself, whether it is a feeling, an experience, or a particular achievement. More important, don't be shy about working on it, shooting high, asking for help, and using everything you can to get there and to make your dreams come true. Once you give yourself goals and set yourself firmly on the path of meeting them, change starts happening, and you can't help but succeed.

So it's time to make that happen. It's time to get going on the seven keys. It's time to unlock secrets that will lead to some incredible, lasting changes in your life. Are you ready? Let's get to it!

Chapter 4

Key 1: Right Thinking

Why You Need This Key:

To change your self-talk so that it's positive and true. This will help you treat your body better and reach your goals.

All you could hear was a whimper coming from beneath the comforter on Kimmie's bed. Tonight, just like so many nights before, Kimmie was lying under the covers in her bed, hiding, and hoping that no one would hear her sobbing. All she wanted was to not have to go to school in the morning. For Kimmie school was hell. It was miserable.

Every day, Kimmie was tormented by a bully. That bully told her she was a disgusting slob with no self-control, insulting her by saying, "You're so fat. You look so gross in that outfit. You're such a loser." But this bully wasn't another guy or girl at school. This bully was Kimmie herself—and she was beginning to believe her own horrible messages. Kimmie had talked herself into believing that she was some kind of loser, and her self-esteem was crashing as a result. Every time she went to school and walked around with her friends (who were all skinny), she would start saying these negative things to herself.

Bully Thinking

As Kimmie found out, the worst bully in your life right now may be you. Do you ever call yourself ugly, fat, a loser, or a failure, or tell yourself you can't do something? All of this—the negativity, the self-criticism, the lies you tell yourself—it's all expressed in the form of an internal dialogue, or "self-talk." Self-talk is that inner conversation you constantly have with yourself, about everything that's going on in your life; it's what you say to yourself in your head that no one else can hear. Sometimes, it is healthy, positive, and factual—what I call "right thinking." But a lot of the time, it is what I call "bully thinking."

Bully thinking has many different angles. Let me list a few of them for you:

- Giving yourself labels like "I'm ugly" or "I'm a whale."

- Assuming you know that people are thinking bad things about you.

- Predicting that you will fail at something. And telling yourself that you are a loser.

- Blaming other people for your troubles, or refusing to take responsibility for changing. For example, blaming your mom for buying candy and leaving it in the kitchen.

- Comparing yourself to other people and deciding you're inferior.

- Telling yourself that you will *never* lose your extra weight or kick your eating disorder.

- Telling yourself that you are not special.

If you are bullying yourself in your own mind—which destroys self-esteem, self-confidence, and self-inspiration—then you're definitely going to have trouble reaching your goals. What if you are getting ready to change your eating habits, or start an exercise program, and your inner bully starts saying things like "I'll never lose weight" or "I'm not going to be able to stick to it, so why even bother?" Then what do you expect will happen to your motivation when you try to improve yourself?

Bully thinking can make you feel inadequate and unable to make important changes and decisions, or cause you not to follow through on your goals. If you see yourself as a loser, you will be a loser. If you predict you're going to fail, you will fail. It is that simple. That sort of negative thinking is sure to drag you down. You end up being your own worst enemy.

In high school it would always just infuriate me when my teammates would hang around the locker room and say that we were going to lose because the other team was way better. I told them this then, and I will repeat it to you now: If you think that you will fail, then you have virtually ensured your failure. So, let's talk about how not to do that.

Your Personal Truth

The problem with bully thinking is that it slowly and silently poisons your "personal truth." Your personal truth is what you believe about yourself—how smart you are, how attractive and self-confident you are, really everything about you. It is how you personally define yourself. It is the truth you live every day as you go out into the world. Your personal truth may be a positive, accurate truth, or it may be a train wreck of lies, distortions, and negative beliefs. If you've ever wondered why you keep shooting yourself in the foot every time you try to improve yourself or your life, it's probably because you tell yourself that you are a hopeless case who will never succeed. If you say those kinds of things, then your personal truth has become one of failure and it sets you up for what your outcome will be.

When your personal truth is out of whack, you tend to take

wrongheaded actions that only make things worse. If you continue to believe lies you tell yourself, put yourself down, think that you'll fail, or give up too easily, you are going to lose confidence in yourself and feel that you're not good enough to reach your goals. You are going to live that mistaken "truth." On the other hand, if you're confident, self-assured, and believe you have self-control, your success will be the result of those perceptions. This phrase sums it up pretty well: What you believe about yourself in your head, is what you will live.

This personal truth business is really, really important to everything we'll be doing in this book—which is why we're starting with this key. What you believe about yourself helps get you to your goals. If you don't get this straight, you'll just keep messing up. You don't want that, and neither do I.

But when you challenge all the self-talk that holds you back, things will change. You will change. You'll be able to go after your goals with confidence and assurance. Your "personal best" will get better and better because what you believe on the inside—your personal truth—is moving you toward new levels of success.

Change Comes from the Inside Out

With this key, you're going to delete your bully thinking and insert right thinking. When this happens, you change yourself from the inside out—so that being fit and healthy is as natural and as normal as breathing. This is important. If all you did was stop eating junk food, you'd make some progress, but that wouldn't last very long because you would not have cleaned up your personal truth. For healthy weight management, change must come from within you. This is where the real power to create lasting results is found. What you are about to do here will give you that power.

Listening to Your Self-Talk

Does your self-talk contain bully thinking? If so, it's important to really tune into it. You need to take a really hard look at what you're telling yourself, day in and day out. In this section you are going to listen to what you're telling yourself about your weight, your body, your appearance, and your self-control (how well you keep yourself from doing the unhealthy stuff). It can feel a little weird to try to hear what's going on inside your head at first, but believe me, it's in your best interest.

Read through the following statements. Do you find yourself identifying with any of them? If any of these statements play in your head, circle *Y* for yes. If a statement does not, circle *N* for no.

Y N   I'm fat.

Y N   I'll never lose weight, or I'll never get over these eating problems or this disorder.

Y N   Everybody thinks I'm fat.

Y N   Only when I get thin will I be happy.

Y N   I blew my diet, so I might as well just eat anything I want.

Y N   I gained two pounds. I knew I couldn't stay thin.

Y N   I wish I looked like ___.

Y N   I'm a failure.

Y N   I hate my body.

Y N   She/he looks better than me.

Y N   I'm so lazy. I can't stick to an exercise program.

Y N   They don't like me because I'm fat.

Y N   My (thighs, hips, stomach, or other body part) is/are too fat.

Y N   If I try (sports, exercise, or other physical activity), I'll fail at it.

Y N   I can't believe I look so bad in (shorts, a bathing suit, jeans, or other clothing).

Y N   I'm disgusted with my appearance.

Y N   I can't stop eating.

Y N   I missed a few workouts. I ruined everything, so I might as well quit.

Y N   I hate exercising.

Y N   Throwing up makes me feel: better, in control, etc. . . . .

Y N   If I'm not on a diet, I'm not taking control of myself.

Y N   People who are thin get more dates.

Y N   People are staring at me because I'm fat.

Y N   I need food to relieve my stress.

This isn't a a test, so there's no grading on this little quiz. I just want you to try to listen very carefully to the statements you've marked—the ones that sound familiar.

Maybe there are other statements running through your mind that are part of your self-talk. Here's how to find out. In the spaces below, write down what you tell yourself about these topics. Write down the positive statements, as well as the negative ones. This is very important because until you know what you are saying, you won't be able to change it.

Use the spaces below, or write your responses in your journal.

Your appearance:

_____
_____
_____
_____

Your body:

_____
_____
_____
_____

Your weight:

_____
_____
_____
_____

Your exercise or activity level:

_____
_____

_____

_____

Your self-control:

_____

_____

_____

_____

Look back over what you've written. Circle any negative statements. Singling out the negatives you tell yourself is a great way to discover things about yourself. When you do this, you expose these negative ideas for what they are—distorted perceptions. Would you say these things to your best friend? No way. So why would you say them to the person you're supposed to care the most about—you!

Now that you have identified these statements, you cannot just take them as the truth anymore. You have to challenge them. Okay, what we just did is a major step toward ensuring your success. Don't forget this stuff, because we are going to discuss it again later.

Action Steps:
The Whole Truth and
Nothing But . . .

Self-talk is what you say to yourself inside your own head. No one hears it but you. That's good—it means that no one can control it except you!

So how do you do it? How do you overcome bully thinking and start believing in yourself and what you can accomplish? How can you avoid a failure mind-set and begin to change yourself from the inside out?

Let me suggest the following three action steps: Test and challenge your bully thinking, replace it with right thinking, and then practice right thinking.

Step 1: Test and Challenge Your Bully Thinking

I'm in law school right now, so I'm learning a lot about how to challenge the truth of someone's testimony by looking at the evidence. You can do the same thing with your bully thinking. Like a prosecutor in a courtroom, you have to put your thoughts on the witness stand and see how they stand up to the facts. In other words, you have to get really picky about your self-talk by asking yourself four simple questions, what I call the Truth Test:

Is what I'm telling myself really true?

Is my thinking hurting or helping me?

Is this way of thinking getting me more of what I want?

If my negative thinking is true, then what do I need to do to change?

Is It Really True?

Most of us don't even question the truthfulness of our negative thoughts, so our self-talk just keeps droning on, wrecking our self-worth and self-confidence. You have to ask if there's any real proof behind your thoughts. What's the evidence for or against your thinking?

Josh, 16, is self-conscious about his weight. He goes around thinking, "No one likes me." *No one,* Josh? Really?

Josh needs to test the accuracy of his self-talk by asking himself these questions:

How do I know people don't like me?

Who do I know who really likes me? (He might list all the people who do like him.)

If there are people who like me, then how can it be true that "No one likes me"?

Josh assumes he knows what people are thinking without having any real proof to back up that assumption. He doesn't know what goes on in other people's heads any more than they know what's going on in his. Life isn't some psychic hotline where we all have the ability to read other people's minds. It's impossible to know what other people are thinking. Even if they are thinking they don't like you, the truth is that worrying about it is just a waste of energy, because you can't control other people's thoughts anyway. You can only do something about yours. And when *you* really start liking you, it won't matter so much what other people are thinking. I love what my dad always says about this: "You wouldn't worry so much about what people thought of you if you knew how seldom they did." Josh needs to get real and stop obsessing over what other people think of him. It is incorrect and it is not helping him.

To Sara, who's 17, gaining a few pounds is "horrible." If Sara were to test that thought by asking "Is it true?" a loud buzzer would go off in her head. Of course, it's not true. It's an exaggeration. "Horrible" is being in a car wreck, or finding out someone close to you is very ill.

If your negative thoughts don't pass this Truth Test, get rid of them. They're lies and they're hurting you. Don't con yourself into believing bad things without cross-examining them. Right thinking is based on what's real—evidence and facts.

Is My Thinking Just a Bunch of Excuses That I Make to Protect Me from the Possibility of Failure?

Sometimes we hang on to self-defeating thoughts because there's a payoff, or advantage, for doing so. When you think, "If I take up tennis, I won't do well," you give yourself a handy excuse for not getting active or trying something new. It's easier to stay in your comfort zone than to reach for something more. But while it may be easier in the short term, you're really selling yourself short. You may even like whatever it is you're talking yourself out of doing once you finally try it!

Or maybe you blame your situation on others. Aaron, 18, tells himself, "My parents are the reason I'm fat." He's convincing himself someone else is the source of his problem, and he refuses to take responsibility for improving himself. He gets to let himself off the hook. That's his payoff. The problem is, until Aaron gets real, he won't be able to make any positive changes.

Then there's Lara, who's 17. She is absolutely convinced in her mind that if she goes out, everyone there will be secretly judging her, thinking how fat she is. So Lara's decided that she won't go out anywhere with anyone until she loses weight. She stays at home, night after night, weekend after weekend, because she is afraid of what everyone else will say about her weight. She believes that by avoiding the situation altogether, she is protecting herself from a lot of hurt and humiliation. But this attitude isn't truthful or helpful. By thinking this way, she's just traded the unhappiness of possible teasing for the unhappiness of being lonely. Lara is getting a payoff—protection from teasing—but at what cost? The lonelier she gets, the more depressed she gets, and the more she eats. Until she confronts the truth, she may never, ever have a chance to be the amazing person she's capable of being.

Are you hiding from the truth, making excuses, or blaming others for your life? If so, how is this kind of thinking really going to help you get in shape or stay healthy? Do your thoughts make you feel happy, calm, peaceful, or motivated? Are they serving your best interests?

If you answered no, no, and no, then stop listening to justifications and excuses that are not working for you. If it's not working, get rid of it.

Is Your Thinking Improving Your Chances of Success or Limiting You Before You Ever Even Start?

To answer this question, you need to think about the goals you set in the previous chapter. What are your goals? Is your self-talk helping you reach them?

Dory, 17, would really like to lose 15 pounds. That's her goal. But her self-talk is full of "I can't" messages: "I can't lose weight." "I can't stick to an exercise program." "I can't stop eating junk food." Her *can't-do's* have overpowered her *can-do's*.

When Dory says to herself, "I can't lose weight," any energy she could have applied to losing weight or staying with an exercise program goes to stressing over how incapable she is, leaving her frustrated and discouraged. She begins to think of herself as a failure before she even begins and sees everything going wrong. Her mindset is focused on failure. Essentially, Dory decides she will fail, and true to that prediction, she fails. But honestly, Dory didn't fail because she couldn't lose weight (she can). She failed because she made her prediction come true. Concentrating on failure assured her failure. When you think the way Dory thinks, don't be surprised when your predictions come true, even if they work against you. An old saying sums it up perfectly, "What you fear, you create."

Like a lot of teens, 14-year-old Jessie wears a self-imposed "fat" label. When she was little, her father used to warn her that she was getting "fat." The label stuck, even though it reflected her father's judgment and not the truth. But Jessie let herself be limited and held back by the label. She let it influence her choices and behavior. She started obsessing over her weight and started a vicious circle of dieting and bingeing, and purging. Fat became a boundary she couldn't get past.

Self-labels limit you because you will live up—or should I say down—to your label. When you stick a negative label on yourself, or when you believe one someone else has slapped on you, you're telling yourself those low expectations are the only ones you should have. Challenge that view of you. If it's unhelpful and untrue, lose the label.

Gail, age 15, is always judging her body, and her inner report card is only a D– on a good day. She thinks her thighs are fat and wishes she looked like a Victoria's Secret model. As long as Gail keeps holding herself up to such unrealistic standards, she may not ever be happy with how she looks or who she is.

Reminder: Self-talk that involves constant comparison is never a good thing. Suppose you decide you need to weigh the least of all your friends. What happens when you become friends with someone who's even thinner than you are? Do you have to lose more weight every time that happens? Comparing yourself to others, and trying to measure up, is a tug of war you can't win. You'll go back and forth, liking yourself one day and hating yourself the next. You feel confident today, but beaten down tomorrow, because you're basing your happiness on something you can't control—someone else's weight or body or looks. Who wants to live like that? The only comparison you should make is, Are you better than you were yesterday? And the only ideal you should live up to is what you know you're capable of achieving. Your goal should be to get to the best possible version of you.

Once you ditch thoughts and labels that stand in your way, you'll be in the fast lane instead of stuck in the driveway.

If My Negative Thinking Is True, Then What Do I Need to Do to Change?

Suppose you've challenged your thinking, and some of your thoughts are true. You've said to yourself that you're overweight, and maybe you *are* because your family doctor said so. Or you told yourself you have gained some weight, and you find out you're three sizes bigger than you were last year. So the statement "I'm overweight" is true. Well, if it's true, then it is a great discovery. Use it to make important changes.

When I was growing up, my dad told me, "Life rewards action." It felt as if he said that at least a thousand times a month. What he meant is that with everything in life, you get only the things you work for. If you do nothing, you will get nothing. Life rewards action.

So if you're sitting at home with 50 pounds to lose, you can start taking steps toward getting out of that situation. You can make an effort to lose weight by getting the information you need, learning positive behaviors, and applying the right tools. Everything you'll learn in these seven keys will help you make the changes you need in order to get the results you want. You have taken a huge step just by getting and reading this book, and that is great. Now, it is time to start using the tools that you are currently picking up as you read along.

You are the only person who can change your life. If you want change, you're the one who can take the action to get you there. No one else can do it for you. If events in your life begin to flow differently, that will be because you have changed what you think, feel, and do.

Step 2: Replace Bully Thinking with Right Thinking

We've looked at a lot of examples of negative, self-defeating, and untrue self-talk in this key. That kind of thinking is a ticket to Nowheresville. You've got to trade it in for right thinking. When you do, the behavior that flows from your "right thinking" will help get you to your goals and help you be a success. Here's what I mean.

Having been involved in sports since I was a little kid—basketball in elementary school, junior high, and high school, and more recently golf—I've been very blessed to have a number of coaches, including my dad, who taught me the importance of the mental side of athletics.

The very first golf instructor I ever had once told me, "If you miss your first putt on the green, never say to yourself: 'Don't miss the next one,' or 'I can't miss my second putt.' " His reasoning was, you don't want the last words you process before you make your second putt or shot to be "don't" or "can't." Instead, he said, tell yourself, "Make the next putt," a much more positive suggestion. He told me: "You choose what you do by what you say to yourself." He was totally right. You do what you say. His advice was centered on the power of suggestion. And as I discovered, it worked.

So now, whenever I play golf, I listen to my self-talk to make sure that my statements are positive and realistic. Whenever I'm playing, I find myself saying things like "I can make this shot. I'm good enough to do this. I can do it." By doing this, I'm plugging positive instructions into my brain. Then the parts of my brain that control how my muscles move take it from there. I'm less likely to slice, duff, or hit the ball into a water hazard. (I know I'm getting some clueless looks right now, but those terms all describe things you *don't* want to do when it comes to golf!)

Let's face it: I'm not playing on the PGA Tour. I'm a college kid trying to get my law degree. I use my inner conversations to put things in perspective. I'm going to have a good time, good game or bad, hit the shower, eat dinner, and start working on a paper for my American Legal History class. That is now, but remember my rule when I was playing basketball in high school? Don't ever say "We are going to lose."

Sports psychologists have known for a long time that the thoughts we have about how we are going to perform a physical activity determine how well we actually do it. Just about every athlete in any sport knows that using self-affirming thoughts can make them winners. All this is completely true for you too, in everything you do. That's why my coach taught me what he did about my thinking. It's the reason I took his advice about what I tell myself on the golf course. I'm no Tiger Woods, but this stuff works for you and me, just as it does for him or any other great athlete. It propels them—and you—toward success.

Before moving on, let me tell you what right thinking is not. Right thinking is not some personal pep rally where little cheer-leaders inside your head shout "Let's be winners!" Changing your self-talk isn't just about the power of positive thinking, or getting rid of every negative belief you'll ever have. Earlier I explained that some of your negative self-talk may be true. If it is, you have to deal with it, and figure out what you need to do to change. The key is to make your self-talk truthful. Then be positive about it. It is al-most as bad to con yourself into thinking that everything is great when the truth is that everything is a real mess. Be optimistic but be truthful to and about yourself.

But when your self-talk isn't true, when it doesn't help you, when it's standing between you and your goals, then it's time for you to energize your thinking and do something different. Choose what's true and what will work. Override bully thinking with right thinking. Here are a bunch of examples that show you how to do what I'm talking about.

Bully Thinking	Right Thinking
I'm a failure.	I've succeeded at lots of different things in my life. I can succeed here.
I can't lose weight.	As long as I do what needs to be done, I'll meet my goals.
I've missed too many workouts. I'll just quit.	Quitting won't get me anywhere. I'll change my schedule to make exercise a priority.
I've gained two pounds, and that's terrible.	I'll think about my week and see where I can do better.
I hate my thighs.	I am learning to love my body and how I feel and look.
I can't have fun anymore if I always have to watch my weight.	Not true. The fitter I get, the more fun I have and the more activities I can do. Life is more fun this way.
I want to look like _____.	I have set goals to help me be the healthiest I can be.

When I get thin, I will be happy.	I won't put off being happy. I will enjoy my life now and work confidently toward my goals.
My parents are making me fat.	I take responsibility for my choices and for changing myself.
Bingeing is the only way to relieve stress.	There are other things I can do to relieve stress, like exercising or talking to my friends.
I have to be perfect.	There is no such thing as perfect. I will cut myself some slack and love myself for what and who I am.

Are you beginning to get the picture? Now it's your turn. Look back at the yes/no quiz you took at the beginning of this chapter and at the statements you wrote about yourself in your journal. Review those messages and test them. Select the ones that are self-defeating, untrue, and negative. Transfer those to the worksheet on the next page, under the column marked "Bully Thinking."

Next, for each bully thought you had, write down an alternative thought in the column marked "Right Thinking." These thoughts should be true, positive, rational, and supportive of your goals. Right thinking will help you live by truths that help you be your best.

Bully Thinking **Right Thinking**

_____

_____

_____

_____

_____

_____

_____

_____

_____

Step 3: Practice Right Thinking

The right thinking you just listed will help you have self-talk that's true and supportive, that will boost your self-control and self-confidence to new levels—as long as you keep using it. The more attention and focus you give this, the more successful you will be at reaching your goals.

You have to understand that changing your thinking is not a one-shot deal; it is a process. You have to always keep working at changing your thoughts and making them more positive, realistic, and constructive. Should bully thinking ever creep into your head, you have to challenge those thoughts, override them, and change them to right thinking to avoid self-sabotage. If you don't keep confronting your inner bully over and over, your thinking and attitude won't change very much, so neither will your behavior. You'll end up getting your butt kicked—by your own beliefs. So stop being so hard on yourself!

Sometimes it helps to refocus your thinking so that you're not dwelling so much on the negative, distorted messages. I remember when I was a little kid and my brother was saying something that I didn't want to listen to. I'd put my hands over my ears and keep repeating, really loud, "I'm not listening! I'm not listening! I'm not listening!" You can do the same thing, mentally. If you do not like it when you have bully thoughts, simply stop listening to them. Focus your thoughts elsewhere. If you are thinking about how much fun you'll have on spring break, then your brain can't dwell on all the things you think are wrong with your life.

The more you do this, the more momentum you'll gain and the more right thinking will become a part of who you are and what you project to the world. When your self-talk is up-lifting, there is a corresponding positive mental and physical energy that rises to the surface. Your self-confidence and regard for yourself will become obvious in your conversations, in the way you look, and in the way you live. Your entire way of being in the world will be different. Got to get in better shape? You will. Win a race? You bet. Overcome problems with eating? Know it and believe it.

As you begin to think differently, you will succeed and you will maximize your life. If you challenge your self-talk, replace it with truth, and live that truth, you will have the inner strength to achieve what you want. You will be much more likely to succeed. So, I have a few questions for you, but don't worry too much. I will even tell you what the answers should be:

Q: What if this plan gets hard?

A: Nothing is too hard for me.

Q: But don't your parents control your meals?

A: They have a huge influence, but I am in control.

Q: You have never been able to do this before. Do you really think that this time is any different?

A: Yes! This time I have a plan and a new set of tools that will program me to succeed. This time it is going to work!

That is how the conversation should go. So, are you finally ready to succeed and take control of your weight once and for all? (You have to answer this one on your own.)

Action Plan

"Right thinking" is a mental frame of mind that says you like yourself and you are a winner. You don't put yourself down, and you don't compare yourself negatively to other people. Right thinking is a healthy attitude that sets you up for success and makes you feel better about yourself and what you can accomplish.

- Listen carefully to your self-talk today, and zero in on your most negative thoughts. Maybe they have to do with your body or a part of your body you think is flawed; appearance; weight; your social life, family, or schoolwork.

Most of my negative self-talk focuses on:

_____

The negative self-talk I use most:

_____

How to change it:

_____

- Sometimes self-talk is true, even if it's negative. If something is true about you that you can change— change it! You get only the things you work for.

Three things I need to change:
1. _____
2. _____
3. _____

What I need to do to change them:
1. _____
2. _____
3. _____

- If our self-talk is mostly negative, sometimes we downplay or disregard things like compliments. Don't do that. Keep a "compliment log" in your journal. Any time someone pays you a compliment, write it down in your journal. Reread your log frequently.

- The best compliments, though, are the ones you give yourself.

What I like most about me are:

_____

- Make a deal with yourself that you will give yourself at least two compliments every day. Write them down in your compliment log too. Or write them on some Post-it notes and stick them up on your mirror so you see them every day.

When you stop putting yourself down, you're going to feel so much more confident and focused on things that count. It takes practice to be a "right thinker," but eventually right thinking will become a part of who you are.

One more thing: With this attitude, you're going to attract a lot of new friends too. People who are positive and upbeat are just naturally popular and fun to be around.

Chapter 5

Key 2: Healing Feelings

Why You Need This Key:

To stop overeating, bingeing, or purging in response to stress or emotional pain.

t's no big mystery of the universe that everybody, especially teens, is under way too much pressure these days. If you are anything like most teens, you're juggling schedules on your PalmPilot, worrying about your appearance and your relationships, dealing with demanding parents, or working toward early admission to college. These days even school doesn't feel safe anymore.

With all of this going on, you may feel as if your life is spinning out of its orbit. Maybe a lot of the time you're stressed out, depressed, fearful, angry, or in the grip of other negative emotions. To complicate matters, you feel out of control a lot of the time because your hormones are running amok and your brain is rewiring itself.

Like a lot of teens, you may do irrational and destructive things when under stress. You might do drugs, withdraw from social life, rebel against any authority, or get into trouble, and on top of all of that you are probably turning to food as a drug to cope with all of the stuff we just listed.

Let's push the pause button on that last one. Because we're talking here about weight issues, our focus in this key will be on how to stop soothing or medicating yourself with food. A lot of us are emotional eaters—that is, we use food as a drug to get through the pressures of life. Or maybe instead of dealing with bad situations by turning to food, we might use food to celebrate. Anytime something good happens we break out the cake, cookies, ice cream, anything sweet. And yes—you guessed it—that makes us overweight, unhappy, and out of control. If you are using food for reasons other than nutrition, which we all do, then we are going to deal with that problem right here in this chapter.

It is perfectly okay to enjoy what you eat and to enjoy eating it. However, what you've got to do is stop self-destructing with food and stop turning to food when you self-destruct. This key will show you how. You'll learn to quit eating your way out of stress and get focused on what really counts. Understand here that I am not trying to suggest that you are an emotional train wreck and that your life is out of control. Now it might be, and if so, we will deal with that here and throughout the rest of this book. But the fact is, we all abuse food to some degree, and for that reason, we all need the info provided in this key. Everybody has emotional issues; everybody abuses food in some way. So pay attention; this chapter is really important for everyone.

The first step toward making a positive change is to acknowledge what you do and how you act when you feel stressed, sad, depressed, angry, or otherwise out of sorts. Let's do that now.

Do You Use Food to Cope?

Let's acknowledge whether you're an emotional eater. In the quiz below, check off the reasons you eat. Please be super-honest in your answers.

Reason	Frequently	Occasionally	Never
1. I munch when I get bored.	( )	( )	( )
2. I like to eat with my friends, even if I am not hungry.	( )	( )	( )

Reason	Frequently	Occasionally	Never
3. I eat so my mom won't be offended.	( )	( )	( )
4. I eat when I get depressed.	( )	( )	( )
5. I eat when I am lonely.	( )	( )	( )
6. I eat when I get anxious about something.	( )	( )	( )
7. There are times when my eating is out of control.	( )	( )	( )
8. I will eat my way through a difficult time (like a breakup, an argument with a friend, a disappointment, or a broken dream).	( )	( )	( )
9. I eat when I feel my energy go down.	( )	( )	( )
10. I crave some foods.	( )	( )	( )
11. I like to celebrate with food.	( )	( )	( )
12. I think about food a lot of the time.	( )	( )	( )
13. I have a tendency to binge.	( )	( )	( )
14. I am embarrassed sometimes by how much I eat.	( )	( )	( )
15. I eat to relax myself and relieve stress.	( )	( )	( )
16. I get upset if I overeat.	( )	( )	( )
17. I eat because I get angry.	( )	( )	( )
18. I hate my weight, but I overeat anyway.	( )	( )	( )
19. I need high levels of sugar in my system.	( )	( )	( )
20. Eating is my main enjoyment in life.	( )	( )	( )

Scoring

For each "frequently" you checked, give yourself 2 points. For each "occasionally," give yourself 1 point, and for each "never," give yourself 0 points. If your score is between 10 and 30, you struggle with emotional eating at times. If your overall score is more than 30, it's likely that you have serious trouble with emotional eating. Acknowledging these things gives you the power to start changing them. So let's get started on that.

The Real Reason Why We Get Upset

If you're like everyone else, you probably think that someone or something upsets you. Your boyfriend dumps you; your parents announce that they're divorcing; you flunk your science test. And so, you get depressed, mad, or anxious, and eat your way through a quart of chocolate chip ice cream.

Here is the catch. The real reason you get upset is not the stressful situation. It's your perception of the situation—how you see it. Everyone sees things differently—very differently. If you are ever to get emotional control, you have got to remember this important law of life: *There is no reality, only perception.*

What I mean by this life law is that our emotions—like unhappiness, fear, anger, anxiety, or depression—are based upon our perceptions of what is happening to us. The interpretations that we make of the events of our lives, and the reactions we have to them, are all that matters. In other words, no matter what happens in your life, how you interpret those events is up to you. For example, some people hate being late, and if they are, it is really stressful for them. Others couldn't care less if they are late. Same event, totally different perception.

If you don't think this life law applies to you, then think about the last time your boyfriend or girlfriend didn't call you on the phone or answer your texts. You immediately start trying to interpret to yourself what not getting a phone call or texts means. Is your boyfriend giving you the cold shoulder? Is your girlfriend getting ready to dump you? Was that person on a date with someone else? Doesn't that person like you anymore?

The next thing you notice is a feeling of depression, fear, or anger. You think that not getting the call or the texts is what hurt you. Actually, it was your thoughts about this event that caused you pain. It's never really the person or the situation that upsets you; it's your perception about it that hurt. You don't react to what happens to you, but you react to your interpretation of what happens to you.

You are probably saying "Uh, Jay, so what?" Well, good question. Keep reading and you'll see.

Filters

Everyone interprets encounters and events through "filters." Filters are like sunglasses. They let some things flow in, but screen other things out. Now, there is an obvious difference in that our filters are not something we can take on and off, like we can with sunglasses. Our filters are internal and mental; they're our personality, attitudes, beliefs, values, points of view, or past events in our lives. They powerfully influence the interpretations we give to situations in our life.

These interpretations, in turn, determine how a person will respond. Have you ever heard the old saying "He sees everything through rose-colored glasses"? This saying is basically talking about someone who has a very positive filter. There are lots of filters that you could have, and while we can't take these filters off like a pair of glasses, we can change our filters, and that is one of the things that we are going to focus on in this chapter.

Having filters is neither good nor bad; it just is. Some filters may be healthy. But many times, these filters are very distorted rather than clear, self-defeating rather than constructive. They tend to let in the negatives, while screening out the positives.

What are your filters? Just knowing them can be a huge help. Here are several examples of filters that have to do with how we view our bodies and handle weight issues.

Denial Filter

This filter causes you to distort certain realities about your body. You tell yourself that you aren't really overweight, but you huff and puff in gym class and can't keep up with everyone else. Or you tell yourself you don't really have anorexia, even though your family doctor says you're dangerously underweight. Denial is a really dangerous filter. Pretending a problem doesn't exist is the fastest way to make it hang around in your life. The emotional pain that comes with the problem hangs around too.

Approval Filter

This filter causes you to make changes in your life based on what other people think of you. You put on makeup so the guy in your math class will like you. You go on a diet because all your friends want to lose weight and you want to fit in. You're relying on other people's approval to validate yourself. If you don't get that approval, you're apt to get depressed or upset and give up on yourself.

Having fun in groups, fitting in, and keeping up with the new styles is perfectly okay. Being a slave to what other people want is not. If you have this filter, it is time to start taking it off.

Perfectionist Filter

This filter causes you to set impossible goals. When your goals are realistically out of reach, then you start viewing yourself negatively and feeling down if you fail to achieve them. You totally measure your self-worth on whether you can meet the perfectionistic standards you have set for yourself.

You may be in great shape, but that's not enough. In fact, nothing is ever enough. The fact is, perfection does not exist, so if you are wearing this filter, it is time to smudge the lenses and move on.

Pessimistic Filter

This is a filter in which everything that happens to you is seen as a catastrophe. You make a melodrama out of every event or encounter in your life. Nothing is ordinary to you. Every pound you gain is the most you've ever gained. Every slip-up you have or mistake you make is a disaster. You can start feeling really angry or frustrated with yourself. Seeing life through this filter has to be miserable. Take it off!

Comparison Filter

This filter causes you to relate to people in a comparative way. You are totally tuned in to what your peers look like and what models in the media look like versus how you can maximize your own God-given body. You measure your self-worth on what your body looks like versus how the bodies of other people look.

I've already talked about the fakeness of media images. But I've got to drive this point home again: Hollywood stars are so airbrushed and taped up (yes, they actually tape body parts to make them look better under clothes), and I have seen them use so many different slimming lenses and lighting techniques to make people look skinnier, stronger, and more fit, that we will never achieve that look. What's more, neither will they when they aren't on camera. So, if you are comparing yourself to others, stop. Seriously, stop.

The thing about all of these filters is that they give you a very skewed, distorted view of yourself and your life. But most important, they are all based on choices you have made about how you see the world. There is no person, nor is there any situation, that can hurt or upset you, unless you allow it to. In other words, no matter what happens in your life, how you interpret those events, and react to them, is up to you. The good news is that you can change your filters. When you do that, your old slant on the world will soon get tossed aside, and you'll start seeing life from a clearer, more factual perspective. A new, more truthful perspective will help you stop using food, bingeing, purging, or other negative behaviors as ways to cope with stress.

So remember: *There is no reality, only perception.* This is a life law you can use to heal just about any emotion, including those that have to do with food issues, your weight, your body image—really anything that is eating you.

Action Steps:
Heal Your Feelings

Okay, let's get down to business. What does it take to heal these feelings that are causing stress, pain, and self-destructive behavior? What does it take to keep from turning to food in times of stress? In the five action steps that follow, you'll learn how to manage your emotions and problem-solve your way out of troubled waters. Taken together, these steps will help you stop stressing out so much, unload painful emotional baggage, and find new ways to cope with stress without resorting to food, overeating, or doing other negative stuff.

Step 1: Change Your Filters

This first step will help you incorporate the life law, *There is no reality, only perception,* into action in your life and use it to your advantage, so that you no longer use food as a drug. You can tell yourself right now that you no longer have to live with the "interpretation" you have put on your life because of your filters. All you have to do is make the decision to change your interpretation (your filtered information). When you do that, you'll respond less emotionally to situations.

One way to do this is by challenging your assumptions. Let's say you view life through the Comparison Filter. You're someone who is always comparing your body to pictures of models in magazines—and you find yourself always falling short. (By the way, everybody falls short, including the models themselves. Don't forget: In real life even they don't look like the airbrushed versions of themselves that we see in the magazines. Cindy Crawford was once quoted as saying, "Even I don't look like Cindy Crawford when I wake up in the morning.")

This comparison business can get you into real trouble. You can freak and go on an extreme diet. This diet is miserable so you go off the diet, binge, get depressed, and gain back even more weight. You end up feeling inadequate and insecure and basically like a fat failure.

These emotions begin to define you, unless you challenge your perceptions. Say to yourself, "My belief that magazine models have a better body than I do and that I need to look like that to be attractive is only my perception. It's not reality. The girls in magazines are airbrushed and retouched to look thin and flawless. It's not real. In fact, they really look too thin and border on looking so thin that it is gross. I will not try to copy some unattainable image in a magazine. I will maximize the best of the real me."

Now let's say you view life through the Approval Filter. You are always making changes to fit in, be accepted, and be liked by others. You believe that doing things to gain the approval of other people will make you successful. It is time to challenge that assumption.

If everything you do in life is to please others, that can be a frustrating path. You are placing your self-worth in the hands of other people. You are constantly seeking their approval to keep you motivated. You are struggling for acceptance every day of your life. Choose to take a more realistic approach and do things for yourself. When you do that, you will always succeed. Other people do not deserve the right to define you, so don't let them. Don't give them that power.

If you're going to change your filters, you'll first have to look at how your own point of view affects your perception of reality. In your journal, list five recent instances when you reacted negatively and resorted to negative behavior like overeating, extreme dieting, purging, or something else in order to cope. These could be a first meeting with someone (when you thought the person didn't like you because of your weight), getting a poor grade on a paper (when you got upset, because you should have worked harder on it), not being asked to the prom (because you see yourself as unpopular), or getting yelled at by your parents (when you felt they were being too restrictive).

These are only examples to get you thinking. Think about your own examples and your negative responses. Then consider the possibility that your "reality" is distorted because you experienced it through a negative filter of your own. After each situation, describe an alternative, more positive or supportive way in which you could have interpreted the situation.

Example

Situation: Getting snubbed at school.

A better way to look at it: Anybody who is that rude doesn't deserve my friendship anyway.

Situation: _____

_____

A better way to look at it: _____

_____

Situation: _____

_____

A better way to look at it: _____

_____

Situation: _____

_____

A better way to look at it: _____

_____

Situation: _____

_____

A better way to look at it: _____

_____

With a better perspective you can manage the stress in your life and regain emotional control. Your perceptions are your choice—and your choice only. I don't care if that crush-worthy guy in third period didn't speak to you. I don't care how tough chemistry class is. I don't care if your parents don't understand you. You choose how to respond to your situation, and your response determines your fate, your weight, and your happiness. This will take commitment and courage. But it will change your life.

Step 2: Act, Don't React

Problems, and the stress they produce, almost never resolve themselves; they don't get better with you twiddling your thumbs and doing nothing. So a big part of handling stress is taking action to resolve what's causing it in the first place. You can either sit around and sulk over the situation, or you can make the choice to be self-directed, take action, and adopt a solution-side approach to your life. If it's the string of D's and F's you got on your report card, worrying about it won't satisfy your teachers or your parents. Maybe you have to learn some better study skills or get a tutor after school. If you're feeling left out at school, withdrawing, pouting, and barricading yourself behind a locked bedroom door won't bring you more friends. Maybe you need to learn how to socialize better with people. If you've unleashed anger and hostility at your mom and dad because you broke the rules, then maybe you need to admit you screwed up and mend fences. Don't sabotage yourself by holding on to your anger. Take action; decide that you will now play offense and solve problems instead of defense when you are hammered by the consequences of mistakes and bad situations.

One more thing: None of these situations will get better if you respond by stuffing yourself with uncontrolled amounts of food. Food is not a fix-it-all.

Ask yourself: Do I just react to what's in my face, or do I act? Start making yourself take action to solve problems and improve your life. If you do, you will get the things you want. This is true with everything—getting better grades, getting along better with your parents, getting a date for Friday night, or getting in better shape. Start taking action now and your life will be filled with victories and rewards.

Step 3: Get Emotional Closure

Changing your response to people, encounters, and events will go a long way toward easing the pain in your life. But there are very possibly some grudges you've been holding. You've been hurt, and you feel angry, bitter, resentful, or sad as a result. As I have said, emotions like these may cause you to take refuge in several orders of fries and cheeseburgers, and a couple of milkshakes to wash it all down. More anger: more pounds. More sadness: more pounds.

As unfair as it is for you to have to be carrying the emotional burden of being wronged by someone else, it is even worse for you to also carry around the physical burden of extra weight as a result. So, are you going to continue to let ugly emotions take root in your heart and mind, contaminating all your relationships? Or will you break out of your personal prison and reclaim your place in the world of happy people?

What you want and what you need is "emotional closure." You want to be able to say honestly that you have no unfinished business left with the people who have hurt you. If you have this burning need to go tell them what jerks they are and you just cannot be at peace until you have done that, then you don't have emotional closure. If every day you get up and feel the need to go over and over in your mind what they have done to you and how unfair it is, then you don't have emotional closure.

Can you do it? Can you get emotional closure? Yes—it's not easy, but it can be done.

What you want to shoot for is what I call the "I'm out of here" response—that is the very least you have to do in order to get emotional closure. This response is going to be different for every person in every situation. For example, if someone at school acts snobby to you, maybe your "I'm out of here" response is as simple as writing that person off, knowing that you will never attempt to be friends with him or her again. If the transgression against you is much more serious, then certainly much more is required.

A good example is Susan, age 17, who attended one of my father's Life Strategies seminars many years ago to look for answers to her 200-pound weight problem. When my dad was talking about how to free yourself from an emotional prison, Susan stood up to speak, trembling, with her voice about to break into heavy sobs. I watched from the back row as her story tumbled out. I'm paraphrasing, but it went something like this:

Viewing Options: ➡ view all messages ➡ view all messages ➡ outline view

UNTITLED MESSAGE

I grew up in a home that was dominated by my father who was in the military. At age 42, he retired from active duty because he had a heart attack. He was home all the time. Most kids would love for their dad to be home a lot, but not me. From age seven, I was continually molested by him. He would always take me up on his lap and begin to touch me in ways and in places that I knew were wrong. I never told my mother. She was a very quiet person who followed my father's orders. I could never count on her to back me up.

But I found a way to resist him. I purposely started overeating to gain weight. I got so heavy, he could barely pick me up. One day, he was trying to lift me onto his lap, and all of a sudden, he stopped breathing. The doctor said that he had died of a massive heart attack. It was no one's fault, he said. Just bad health.

Although he's dead and I'm relieved that he no longer walks the earth, I feel locked in an emotional prison of guilt, anger, and bitterness. I feel dirty, ugly, and damaged. I've withdrawn and retreated further into food and bingeing. I'm afraid to date, or even make friends. I am afraid of guys in general. I can't get the memory of what he did to me, and what I did to him, out of my mind.

➡ reply to this message ➡ add to favorites ➡ view all replies

Susan had internalized and was hammering herself each day with the horrible acts committed by her father. They were eating away at her heart and soul. What happened to her was horrible. He should not have stolen so much from the life of this girl. But he had. As long as she remained filled up with anger, bitterness, and guilt toward her father, she would stay locked in a bond with him that would absolutely poison her spirit and she would never ever be able to lose that weight or get on with her life. It is a huge understatement to say that Susan had some major, unfinished emotional business.

My father told everyone in the room that the prison door locks from the inside out. Only we can let ourselves out and control our own lives. What Susan had to do—and what you want to do—is identify the least demanding thing that will allow emotional closure and the ability to move on.

This requires a simple four-step process. When you put it into action, trust me, it will lessen your need to binge and use food as medication. Let's go through it now so you can refuse to live with unfinished emotional business and take your power back.

1. Figure out who in your life has you locked in the tractor beam of painful emotions and hurt. Next to their name(s) describe what it is they have done to you and, therefore, the thing about which you must get emotional closure. _____

_____

_____

2. Search your mind and heart, and identify your "I'm out of here" response. Do you need to confront them? Or can you handle this entirely within you? Do you need

to write them a letter or e-mail? Do you need to call the police? What is the least action you can do that will allow you to say, "This is it. I'm out of here"?

_____

_____

3. Commit yourself to action. Put it in writing here. I commit myself to (describe the action you have decided on): _____

_____

_____

I will do this by (give yourself a real-time deadline):

_____

_____

4. If you are successful at doing this, write the words to describe how you will feel once you are free of the negative emotions that have had you locked in a bond with this person. _____

_____

_____

We heard from Susan after the seminar. Her "I'm out of here" response was to write down all her thoughts and all her feelings in a letter. Because her father was dead, she couldn't send it to him. So she went to the cemetery where he was buried and read it to him at his grave. This might sound crazy to you, but for Susan, it was the ultimate step that she needed to get the pain out of her heart and out of her mind. Susan wrote to my dad when it was over; she felt that a huge burden had been lifted from her life. She was finally free.

Step 4: Tap Into the Power of Forgiveness

There is one other action you can take to get emotional closure, and it's called forgiveness. Another one of my life laws states that *there is power in forgiveness.* The reason is that, without forgiveness, you are destined to hold grudges, anger, and bitterness. You can suffer not only emotionally, but physically too. Holding grudges and staying mad or bitter can make you get sick.

The best thing for you is to forgive. When you forgive people, you thrive in spite of them. You flourish. You realize that as good as it feels to hold a grudge, overcoming a grudge feels a whole lot better.

Does this mean that I'm telling you to go to the person who has hurt you and say "I forgive you"? No way. The forgiveness I am talking about is all about you and not about whoever has hurt you. I don't care if these other people ever even know that you have forgiven them. I don't care if they ever even acknowledge they have hurt you. You are the only person who has to know about this forgiveness because this is something that takes place within you and for you. Forgiveness is a choice, a choice that you make to release yourself from the emotional prison of anger, hatred, and resentment. I am not saying that the "choice" is an easy one, only that it's a must-do one.

If you are unsure as to how to forgive—if you are unsure about what to say within your heart—let me help you give a voice to your choice of forgiveness. You might say the following to yourself:

I choose to forgive you. By doing so, I free myself from the bond I had with you through hatred, anger, resentment, or fear. I take my power back and gain the freedom that only forgiveness can bring. You cannot hurt me, and you cannot control me. I forgive for myself.

Sometimes the person you most have to forgive is yourself. Hanging on to negative feelings about *you* can do as much damage as any anger or resentment you have toward someone else. To get on with your life, you need to forgive yourself and put any mistakes you've made behind you. Forgiving yourself is a must if you want to continue to make positive changes.

You have to let the negative emotions go if you want any chance to heal your feelings. Forgiveness is a great way of cleaning your emotional house. You sweep out all the crap that's cluttering up your life and making it difficult to move forward. By forgiving yourself, and those who have wronged you, you free yourself.

Once you have identified and carried out your "I'm out of here" response from Step 3, this whole forgiveness thing is much easier. The key is to totally release yourself from the bond that you have with the people who have hurt you. Often, forgiving them is the only way to do that. So, let's move on.

Step 5: Cope Without Food

When you're under stress, your nerve cells get restless, and it's not easy to quiet them down. Sure, you can do it quickly by resorting to chemical means such as alcohol, drugs, or high-calorie comfort foods like candy bars, cookies, and ice cream. But those will blow any chance you have of healthy weight management.

A far better way to restore calm and blow off steam is to carve out time in your life for tension-reducing activities. These activities include, but are not limited to, exercising (a powerful stress reliever and my personal favorite!), doing meditative things like yoga, performing relaxation exercises, and listening to music. They work directly on your nervous system by releasing *endorphins,* your brain's tranquilizers, to give you a natural high.

When you consider various tension-reducing activities, I realize that you may not be open to relaxation exercises like deep breathing. Maybe you think they won't help or that they won't work. But what if something like this is exactly what you need when anxiety, stress, or depression hits? What if it is?

I'm not trying to go Super-Weirdo-Guru on you here, but let me tell that I'm a huge fan of breathing. You see, when you feel stressed, your breathing becomes shallow, and this creates more tension. Less oxygen gets to your brain. When your brain is low on oxygen, this triggers feelings of depression. Stress throws you off balance in so many ways.

One of the most effective methods for restoring oxygen and balance is to breathe in a controlled pattern. You simply breathe out for the same amount of time as you breathe in. For example, count to 7 as you exhale and then to 7 when you inhale, repeating the pattern again and again. In less than a minute, the muscles in your body get less tense. Your brain senses this, interprets it, and begins to release endorphins that further reduce the tension level in your body. Pretty soon, your tension is gone, and you're in the realm of relaxation. In fact, I just tried it and almost fell asleep. Of course it is 12:30 a.m., but then again, I am a night owl. Anyway, it really does work.

To help you learn this technique, there is a fun breathing exercise (Supplement A) in the back of the book. Once you make this form of breathing a habit, it becomes a very good tool for keeping your cool during stressful situations—and not caving in to food to calm you down. When you can learn to clear your thoughts and emotions through deep breathing, people and events cannot throw you off balance so easily.

As you incorporate more tension-reducing activities in your life, please continue to work hard on how you react to stress. Change your responses so you don't become unglued. This will help you manage your emotions in the long run. Even so, something as simple as breathing deeply, exercising, or listening to music will help you calm down so that you can at least check your reactions to the stress. That way, your thinking can stay sharp and you will stop drugging yourself with food.

Healed Feelings

Learning to heal your feelings will do two things: It will zap the frequency and intensity of painful emotions. And it will cut down on the number of times you slide back into the old self-destructive patterns of overeating, bingeing, and other actions that mess up your weight control.

When you put these steps into action, you'll love how much more orderly, peaceful, and fulfilling your life gets. You'll have a newfound sense of freedom. You'll feel so much better about yourself and more in control of you.

Action Plan

We all get stressed out and feel down from time to time, and that's okay. But if you continually turn to food and other self-destructive behaviors to make yourself feel better, that's not okay. One of the worst things about emotional overeating is this: You are no longer in control of your life. The self-destructive behavior like overeating or purging is.

With this key, you now have a bunch of tools you can use (instead of food) to help you deal with your problems and not eat emotionally. You can change your filters, work to solve your problems, get emotional closure (the "I'm out of here" response), forgive people who have hurt you (and yourself), and learn how to relax when you're stressed. Practice these things, and little by little, the self-destructive things you used to do will be history.

- List the five biggest things (people, situations, or emotions) that cause you to overeat, binge, purge, or even avoid eating:

  _____

  _____

  _____

  _____

  _____

- Why do these things bug you? What filter do you need to change?

  _____

  _____

  _____

  _____

  _____

- Problems never get solved by doing nothing. Solutions are the result of action. If you've been eating because something is eating you, put together a plan to resolve the problem:

  The problem that's eating me: _____

  My plan for resolving it: _____

- Are you holding a grudge? List your best "I'm out of here" responses.

- Before you go to bed tonight, write a note of forgiveness to someone who has hurt you. (You don't have to mail it unless you want to.)

- Right now if you can, stop what you are doing and practice deep breathing for about five minutes. How did it make you feel?

- List five things you can do that will take the place of overeating when you feel stressed out.

_____

_____

_____

_____

_____

If you will follow and use at least some of the steps we talked about here, you will be amazed at how much better your life will feel. Being able to handle stress and ease tension without resorting to food will give you more time to focus on things like having fun, being with your friends, developing one or more of your talents, doing better in school, or whatever is most important to you. There are lots of ways to treat yourself well, and healing your feelings is one of the best.

Chapter 6

Key 3: A No-Fail Environment

Why You Need This Key:

To set up your world for success, making healthy choices the easy choices.

Andrew is one of my best friends from high school, and during our sophomore year he started to gain weight. By the time we started our junior year, he was way overweight. In fact, he had gained so much weight our football coach told him he needed to slim down. Now think about that, I haven't met too many guys who are *too big* to play football, but somehow Andrew pulled it off.

So, we sat down and figured out how he was going to lose weight and get in better shape. When we first started looking at the situation, it didn't make sense. We figured that maybe he was just a big guy and that there wasn't any way that he could lose weight without going on some major diet.

The thing was, he exercised; his mom made healthy meals; his parents weren't overweight. It just didn't add up (that is, of course, with the exception of his weight, which was really adding up). Well, it didn't take long before we realized why Andrew had gained so much weight. In fact when it dawned on us, we figured out why all of us had packed on a few extra pounds in the last year.

You see, right near our high school, a new ice cream place had just opened. It was one of those places where you pick the flavor of ice cream, pick the toppings you want, and then the person behind the counter mixes it all up for you. We had all started going there after school to hang out. We were eating ice cream every day, and as a result, every one of us started to gain a few extra pounds. I mean, we were hanging out at an ice cream shop. Can you really expect us not to eat a few scoops each day? I didn't think so!

Well, Andrew is a little different story. He didn't go hang out there after school; he worked there after school! He was there every day for hours, often with nothing to do. So he started eating the free ice cream and food he was allowed to eat as an employee. He was there every single day just staring at all kinds of ice cream and with boxes of Butterfingers (before they were broken up and used for toppings) and Coke on tap.

With all of that temptation it was virtually impossible for Andrew to say no. Just as it was impossible for the rest of us to visit him at work and not have some ice cream too. When Andrew realized that he was slowly grazing on all of the stuff at work each day, he decided to quit his job. As soon as he did, we all started to lose some weight, especially Andrew. The problem was that he was spending a huge amount of time in an environment where it was virtually impossible not to eat lots of fattening food.

Saying no was too hard, so he decided to put himself in a different situation where he didn't have to say no. That is exactly what this chapter is all about: creating an environment where you don't have to say no. As we go through this chapter, think back to Andrew and follow his lead for creating a no-fail environment.

So far, you've looked at yourself from the inside out. You've gotten real about how your thoughts and emotions have been sabotaging you. Now it's time to change your focus and look at how your external world—"your environment"—is doing the very same thing.

The other day one of my professors made us go to the library to do some research. So, I did some research. I don't think that she meant that she wanted me to do research for my new book, but hey, she should have been more specific. You know that huge dictionary that nobody ever uses? Well, I used it. I looked up *environment* and here's some of what it said: *the circumstances, objects, or conditions by which one is surrounded; the social and cultural condi-*

tions that influence the life of an individual. In other words: the people you know, the places you go, the things you see, experience, smell, feel, and touch. The world around you, and how it affects you.

A lot of the time, that world is pretty toxic—and I'm not talking about hazardous waste but rather the sense that your environment is spring-loaded with temptation and pressure that can trigger you to do things like overeat or lose unhealthy amounts of weight. You can't successfully manage your weight unless you change things in your external world too. That's what this key is all about.

Remember at the beginning of this book I said that you would not need to rely on willpower because we were going to put your weight on project status?

One of the big ways we are going to do that is set up your world (your environment) so that you are successful. You see, we are going to just assume that on some days you won't want to work toward a healthy body (because that is true of everybody). So we are going to protect you from failure now.

Here's an example of what I'm talking about: If there is no junk food around, then you can't eat junk food. So, we are going to get rid of the junk food and as the title says, create a "no fail environment" for you. If you use this key, I promise that reaching your goals will be a thousand times easier.

This key uses two sayings you've heard a million times (because they're true!). The first is, "Out of sight, out of mind": If there's no 10-pound bag of peanut M&M's waiting for you when you get home from school, then obviously you can't eat them and you probably won't even think about M&M's. You're also much less likely to overeat in general. I mean, who wants to binge on broccoli?

Then there's the other saying: "The right place at the right time." It's much easier to choose a healthy lunch if you're eating at your gym's smoothie shop or some place with a good menu (like home) than if you're at some fast food drive-through or a vending machine. So choose not to go to McDonald's in the first place. Too much undesirable behavior occurs when you put yourself in situations where it is hard to avoid eating badly. It is *much* easier not to order a chocolate shake if you are eating somewhere that doesn't serve chocolate shakes. If you go to a fried chicken place for lunch, then chances are, you are going to eat fried chicken. Instead, go to a sandwich shop because then the chances are that you are going to eat a sandwich. There are too many temptations when you put yourself in situations where it is hard to avoid eating badly.

This key is going to teach you how to create your own no-fail, self-healing, goal-reaching environment. This is an especially important key for you as a teen, because it shows you how to influence different situations in your life. I know you think you don't have any control over things like what you eat for dinner and what food is in the fridge because you live with your parents and they make all those decisions. But that's only true to an extent. You are going to discover that you have a lot more control over your world than you ever imagined. You know the old advice, "Never go grocery shopping when you are hungry"? Well, we are going to go grocery un-shopping while you are not hungry. What I mean is that we are going to get rid of all that junk food *before* it is screaming "Eat me." Like I've said, if it is not there, then you can't eat it.

Trust me, this approach works. Why? It works because changing your environment helps shape your behavior. Changing your environment is one of the best methods of self-control. You can set up your world so that it becomes easy to make healthy choices. That means no relying on willpower!

Those Crazy Things You Do: The Power of Cues

Your environment can make you do dumb things you don't want to do if you let it. That's because it's loaded with "cues." You know what a cue is if you've ever taken drama or been in a school play. It's a signal to do something, like recite a line.

Cues are everywhere. A green light at the intersection is a cue to go; a red light is a cue to stop. A beep on your computer is a cue to read your e-mail; a telephone ring is a cue to answer the call. A hot guy or girl walking by is a cue to check that person out.

Likewise, there are cues in your environment that trigger you to overeat, purge, or do whatever your behavior is. Other cues in your environment, such as the media, get you to think about your body in some very negative ways. All of these cues can scream pretty loud, catching you off guard and making you act or think in ways that go against the goals you've set for yourself. These types of cues can include anything from a TV commercial for cookies to the toy that you got (and that we all wanted) if you ate a Happy Meal.

At other times cues can be really sneaky. You don't ever even realize that they are there, influencing your behavior. For my brother Jordan, every time he smells cut grass, he wants to play baseball. He doesn't think about it, and the cue (smelling grass) is very subtle, but the reaction is very strong. So if you've got problem behavior that you want to change, you want to avoid the cues that trigger it.

Let's get a little more specific about what those cues are. Most cues involve *people, places, things, feelings,* and *senses.*

People

The power of people to influence your behavior is huge. When it comes to food, parents are the people who have the most control over what you eat. They shape your food behavior with the foods they buy and fix for you. They shape your eating habits by making you clean your plate, pacifying you with sweets, or offering food bribes ("If you eat your vegetables, you can have dessert").

If your parents try to micromanage what you eat, practically force-feeding you healthy stuff like Brussels sprouts and beets, that could easily turn into a power struggle. You rebel by eating all the wrong stuff and too much of it. So, maybe your parents' insisting on you eating healthy food is a cue to rebel and eat a bunch of junk food. Or maybe your parents are always on a diet, and being around them is a cue that makes you self-conscious about being or getting fat.

One of the scary things about self-destructive behaviors like overeating, bingeing, dieting, and even abusing alcohol is that they can be passed down from parents to teens. But the good news is it doesn't have to be that way—you can break the pattern and make your life different. As my grandfather always used to say, "You have the power within you to rise above your raising."

Your friends and other teens influence your actions too. You want to fit in, so you do what they do, eat what they eat. Sometimes this is healthy and constructive, but it may also be destructive. I once saw a bumper sticker that explained this perfectly. It said: "Don't follow me. I'm lost too." It sounds funny, but it's actually really smart and totally true. Chances are your friends don't know squat about eating healthy (even if they're good at acting like they do). If you start following others' bad behaviors, you may fall into a rut that can be hard to get out of.

There's nothing wrong with wanting to be with people you like. The problem starts when being around their negative behaviors makes it too hard for you to do things differently. Recognize that cue: If being around your friends makes you want to stuff your face with pizza and ice cream, then maybe you should eat before you go out, so you won't be hungry and tempted to eat too much.

Places

The places you go can be cues that trigger overeating, binge-ing, and other unwanted food behaviors. Fast food restaurants, drive-throughs, food courts, snack bars, parties, movie theaters, convenience stores, and other places where you hang are cues. Places in your house, like where you sit when you watch TV, and even places at school or being in your car are cues too.

Going to restaurants and parties, watching TV, and being with your friends are all an important, healthy part of your life. Hanging out at the mall is a great way to socialize with your friends, for example. But when you do it every weekend, and you can't seem to do it without hitting a Chinese takeout for a few egg rolls, then the mall has become any unhealthy trigger for you.

Right now you are probably saying, "Yeah, Jay, I like hanging out with my friends at the mall and that being a cue to eat doesn't change anything. And chapter two of that story is I'm not going to stop hanging out with my friends." I hope that is what you are saying, and I'm not suggesting differently. Right now, I just want you to identify your cues; we will talk about how to deal with it all a little later.

Things

There are also "things" in your environment that egg you on and influence you to make unhealthy choices—and there are a million of them. There are vending machines, super-sized value meals, ads for food and diets on TV, online, or in magazines (many of which are designed to speak directly to teens). There are also things at school, like all those fundraising drives for the soccer team or National Honor Society where the students sell bags of M&M's or chocolate bars. How can you resist when all that candy is in your face and for such a good reason? And forget it if you're the one selling. Constantly having an entire carton of chocolate by your side is way too tempting for some people. How many times have you been the one to eat half the stuff you're supposed to be selling?

No question about it: It's hard to avoid this kind of stuff. But you can do it. You just have to create your environment so that it supports your goals, and gets you closer to what you want. Remember, right now we are just trying to recognize cues.

Feelings

As you discovered in Key 2, emotions are among the biggest instigators of repeated overeating, bingeing, purging, starving, and other extremes. You can get so bored, so lonely, so depressed, so rebellious, or so down on yourself that you eat your way through the kitchen. Positive emotions can trigger binges too. Whatever emotion you were feeling at the time you started eating was probably a cue. Food is a quick fix that soothes emotions. But as you learned, you control how you respond to what happens to you, and that includes how you react to certain emotions. Maybe feeling sad is a cue to either throw up or eat a gallon of ice cream, or both. If so recognize that.

Senses

The sight, smell, and taste of food are powerful cues that can reel you in. You know this if you have ever been tempted by the smell of a big juicy burger or by a batch of freshly baked cookies. Why do you think they show someone pulling apart a cookie with gooey, melting chocolate in that Toll House commercial? Because just the sight of it is a powerful cue.

Ironically, probably the healthiest and most important "sense" cue for eating is the one that a lot of people with weight and eating problems totally ignore. That cue is hunger. It's pretty amazing how people will eat for every reason except because they're hungry. One way to get your weight under control is eat when you're truly hungry, rather than to eat because of cues like people, places, things, emotions, or the other senses.

Scavenger Hunt: Find the Cues in Your Environment

Looking over what we've just talked about, what cues are at work in your life? Let's begin to find out with the following activity. It will help you pinpoint the environment cues that get to you.

This activity is like a scavenger hunt, only in this case you're searching for cues in your environment. As you look over these categories, ask yourself: Which of these cues triggers me to eat, overeat, binge, purge, go on a diet, or do anything else unhealthy? Under each category, circle or underline all words that apply. If you can think of other cues in each category, list them in the spaces marked "Other."

People:

Best friends	Students in clubs	Sister(s)
Other friends	Parents	Other relatives
Teammates	Grandparents	Seeing fat people
Students in class	Brother(s)	Seeing skinny people

Other people: _____

Places:

Restaurants	Kitchen in your house	Sleep-overs
Fast food places	Dining room in your house	Your car
Drive-throughs	Your bedroom	Someone else's car
Mall food court	Other places in your house	School
Snack bars	Movie theater	Your workplace
Bakery	Games and sporting events	Places you visit
Convenience stores	Concerts	
School cafeteria	Parties	

Other places: _____

Things:

Time of day	School or church fund-raising campaigns or activities	Thoughts or fantasies about food
Vending machines		
Super-sized meals	Exposure to food ads	Any media images, including music videos, that make you feel bad about your body
Music	Posters	
Favorite foods	Internet	
Free or discounted food at work	Prizes at fast food restaurants	
	Colorfully packaged foods	

Other things: _____

Feelings / Senses:

Hunger	Appearance of food	Sadness
Food cravings	Smell	Loneliness
Taste	Emotions	Rejection
Sight of food	Fear	Feeling fat

Other feelings or senses: _____

Once you become more aware of these cues, it's time to take action. Minimizing or getting rid of them is a huge step toward getting and maintaining more self-control.

Action Steps:
Operation Clean Sweep—
Getting Rid of Cues

For healthy weight management, you've got to eliminate as many of these cues as you possibly can, or at least try to avoid them. You've got to put certain cues "out of sight, out of mind," and put yourself in "the right place at the right time." So, now that you have identified all of your cues, let's talk about what to do to protect yourself from those cues.

What follows are seven action steps you can take, starting right now, to get your environment, and consequently your behavior, under better control.

Step 1: Set Up Your No-Fail Environment

Review the cues you circled in the quiz. Are there ways to get food out of sight, out of mind? Can you put yourself in the right place at the right time?

Here are some strategies to help get your brain in gear:

- Arrange activities with your friends that don't include food.

- If you're more prone to problem eating with certain people and you don't want to avoid them, tell them you're trying to eat healthy and ask for their support.

- Practice the art of saying no. If you're caught in a situation where there's peer pressure to do something you don't want to do, just say, "Sorry, guys, I'm outta here."

- Empty all the food out of your purse, your glove compartment, your locker, and all other places you stash food.

- Pack your own healthy meals and snacks to take to school or work.

- Don't take any more money than you really need for school each day; that way, you're less likely to "feed" the vending machines.

- If driving home from school or work takes you by your favorite fast food place, find another route.

- Eat a healthy meal or some healthy snack before you go to a party or other social event. That way, you'll be less likely to pig out later.

- Schedule healthy activities. If the first thing you do when you get home from school is tear into a bag of chips, plan to do something else to avoid your snack attack, like reading a book, exercising, or doing relaxation exercises. (You'll learn more about strategies like this in the next key.)

- Ask your parents if you can donate some of the foods you no longer want to eat to a food bank in your community. (Or find some other way to get the stuff out of your house.)

- Give away the free or discounted food you receive at work to people who aren't dealing with food issues, or donate them to charity.

- Pre-plan what you're going to eat. For example, decide ahead of time what you'll order when you go to a fast food restaurant: grilled chicken sandwich, baked potato, hamburger with lettuce and tomato (no cheese or special sauce!), a sandwich wrap, or a salad. When you don't have to make a decision on the spot, it's easier to make the right decision. And every time you make a good choice, you get stronger, so the next time it becomes easier to make that decision. But if you fail to plan, you plan to fail.

- Consider quitting or switching jobs—like my friend Andrew did. If you have issues with eating and you work at a grocery store, convenience store, restaurant, or other food-related business, you're basically surrounding yourself with powerful cues. That's like being an alcoholic and working in a bar. Why purposely put yourself in situations that are too tempting?

At this point, you're probably ready to muzzle me and say, "C'mon, Jay. It's not that easy."

You're right. Avoiding temptation and pressure is a lot easier said than done. But it is possible. The point is to make little changes where you're the most vulnerable so that your world is geared for success. Believe me, it's a lot easier to avoid triggers than to fight them. And it is easier to stay away than it is to stare right at temptation and say "No thanks."

I've given you a push here; now it's time for you to get rolling. If you want different, you have to do different. And you have to do different by taking major action.

Use what you've learned in this step to list other actions you can personally take to get rid of or avoid the cues you identified in the quiz. Feel free to add to this list as you complete this key.

My action steps for dealing with people:

_____
_____
_____
_____
_____
_____

My action steps for handling places:

_____
_____
_____
_____
_____
_____

My action steps for dealing with things:

_____
_____
_____
_____
_____
_____

My action steps for managing feelings and senses:

_____

_____

_____

_____

_____

_____

Step 2. Develop New Tastes

No one would debate that taste is probably the most powerful food cue. Certain foods just make your mouth water. For me, it's a Dairy Queen Oreo Blizzard. (For those of you who don't know what Dairy Queen is, you really should visit Texas sometime. DQ is what we Texans refer to as the Texas Stop Sign. It is some really good ice cream.) I consider the Oreo Blizzard one of the major food groups. I start salivating just thinking about it. There's no deep, dark reason why I love those things. Oreo Blizzards just taste good—that's all there is to it.

But tastes and preferences for foods can change. Remember when you were a little kid and you used to chug whole milk like it was going out of style? Then, as you got older, you switched to drinking skim milk. At first, it tasted bland and watery, but you kept on drinking it. Eventually you got used to it; then you even started to like it. Now when you drink whole milk, you practically gag because it tastes so heavy and rich.

Shrinks call this *choice shift*. Anytime you replace a food with its healthier version, and keep on eating the healthier one, that healthy food actually begins to taste better to you. This really does happen, I swear.

Try something with me, at least while you're learning these

keys and starting to apply them to your life. Instead of eating regular chips, cookies, candy, or sugary sodas, trade them in for their low-fat or sugar-free versions. (And just because you're eating low-fat *does not* mean you can eat more of them. It doesn't work that way.) Also try adding other foods into your diet, like fresh or dried fruits; fresh vegetables with low-fat dips; low-fat milk products like yogurt or reduced-fat cheeses. See if your taste preferences begin to adjust.

Confession: I'm not sure what I'd eat in place of an Oreo Blizzard. Flavored milk? Yogurt? Dunno. I'll work on that one and get back to you.

Step 3: Eat When You're Truly Hungry

Hunger is the true, healthy cue for eating, the one that tells you how much fuel you need for survival. What happens is this: The hypothalamus (I had to use that word, by the way), a tiny area in your brain that is about the size of a garbanzo bean. (What the heck is a garbanzo bean, you ask? I don't know either, but when I asked, some smart aleck pointed out that all beans are the same size, so basically it is the size of a bean.)

If you're hungry, you might feel a hollowness in your stomach or hear it grumbling. You might get a skull-crushing headache. Or you might feel low on energy, because your blood doesn't have enough blood sugar to nourish your body's cells.

These signs of hunger are meant to be disagreeable so that you will relieve them by eating. Then, about 20 minutes into your meal, your hypothalamus tells your brain that the amount of fuel in your body is just about right and it's time to stop eating. That's why you start to feel full.

You have to recognize and pay attention to these signals. Try to eat when you're truly hungry, and only until you are reasonably full—not gut-busting, "I'm so stuffed I can't move" full. (In Texas we would unbutton the top button of our jeans at that point, and that is exactly what you don't want to do.) Don't ignore your body's call for food. This is one of the seldom-practiced secrets to healthy weight control. But just don't go overboard.

Step 4: Get Your Parents on Your Side

Getting rid of cues takes cooperation from the people in your life, especially your parents. They buy the food. They fix the food. They serve the food. They seem to be in absolute control, but are they?

Yes and no. More teens than ever are now doing the family grocery shopping. Teens going grocery shopping? Better believe it. While most people think that's what moms do, the reality is that more than half of all teenage girls and more than a third of all teenage boys do some food shopping each week. And think about it, if you offered to do the job for Mom, do you think she'd really argue?

But even if you don't shop for groceries, you still influence what your parents buy. Some proof:

- Seventy-eight percent (78%) of teens and children influence where their family goes for fast food.

- Fifty-five percent (55%) of teens and children influence the choice of restaurant for dinner.

- Thirty-one percent (31%) of you have a say in what products your mom buys at the grocery store.

- Teens directly influence nearly $20 billion in grocery purchases made each year. That's a lot of *dinero*. (If it helps, that $20 billion would wrap around the earth almost 79 times if the dollar bills were laid end to end.)

- Most parents, when surveyed, say that their children— not themselves—are the family members most influential in selecting fast food, snack food, and restaurants.

You may not have total control, but you do have the ability to get your parents to do more of what you want to do and less of what you don't want to do. So use the power you do have. Here's how.

Your parents will treat you according to the way you act. If you show them that you really like Brussels sprouts, they will probably start buying Brussels sprouts. Moms love to feed their kids the foods they want—like when your mom insists on making your favorite dinner the first night you come home from sleep-away camp.

Even so, your parents might be resistant at first. Why? Because all along you asked your parents to buy you Twinkies and to drive you to McDonald's for Happy Meals. You've already taught your parents a few things about what you want, and like you, they're used to it. So if there's going to be a change in the routine, it's only fair that you prepare them for what's coming. If you teach someone to play a game, when the rules change, the players are entitled to know so they can adjust their strategy.

I'll talk more about how to build your parents' support in Key 7, but for now, try asking them to buy healthier food. Be calm, and don't make any demands. Just talk to them about your goals. And don't get mad if you don't get the response you want. Tell them about your plan, but most important, show them—prove you're serious with your actions. No matter what their initial reaction is, stick to your goals. That way, you'll inspire confidence and trust.

Your parents react to you. In that respect you are in control of the relationship. When you show them that you really want an apple instead of a Snickers, you teach them that you are serious, predictable, committed to change, and competent. You tell them with your actions.

Step 5: Stop Buying In

U.S. businesses spend millions of dollars *every hour* of every day promoting and advertising food to parents, teens, and kids. They do this by concocting sugary, fatty, and salty foods that can be really addictive. They reel you in by selling super-sized meals at value prices. They tell you that eating it will bring you more fun, happiness, and popularity. When a barely dressed Britney Spears dances on TV while drinking Pepsi, the message is "To be sexy, drink Pepsi."

They want your cash!

If you're like my brother and me, you probably constantly whine to your parents that you have no money, but in reality, teens, as a whole, spend about $140 billion a year, a lot of it on food and snacks.

One fast food value meal a day adds up to $1,500 a year. Imagine how many CDs you could buy with that!

Right now you may be unaware of the forces around you that are trying to get you to eat or to be thin. You're more worried about your fourth-period history test, or who will drive you to the game Friday night. But there's a lot at stake here.

If you continue to let food and advertising industries make your choices for you, then you're giving away your power. You control what you buy or don't buy. You control where you eat or don't eat, and what you decide to eat when you get there. You control your reactions to the advertising blitz.

What I'm calling on you to do is refuse to be taken in by this stuff. Don't believe the hype, and don't buy the crap they're selling.

Step 6: Know Your Enemy

We just spent a lot of time getting to know your cues for negative behavior. Well, they always say that the best way to defeat your enemy is to know your enemy. I agree with that idea. I think that now that you are aware of those cues and their impact, you have a much better chance of stopping that impact.

If you know that going to the mall to hang out *always* leads to you eating pizza and ice cream, then you can prepare for that and change the results without staying home.

Here are some ways to take the power away from your cues to negative behavior:

- Plan ahead: Eat before you go to the mall.

- Change the effect of the cue: Decide that if you go to the food court, you are going to have a salad or a fruit smoothie and nothing else.

- Make a decision that you won't be controlled by cues and make a conscious effort not to cave in.

Step 7: Become an Activist

This one's optional, thrown in for those of you who like circulating petitions and lobbying for stuff you're passionate about. Become an activist—by campaigning for healthier food choices at your school. This involves persuading the people at your school who have the power to do something about the situation. Some tactics to consider:

- Join forces with friends who feel the same way you do; go to your school administrators and say you want healthier foods in the school cafeteria and vending machines. Tell them in addition to French fries and mac and cheese you want a salad bar, or ask for a frozen yogurt machine instead of ice cream.

- Put together a petition drive and get signatures to build support.

- Work with the parent-teacher organization at your school to get teachers and parents on board with the students, because there's strength in numbers.

- Ask that refrigerated vending machines be stocked with low-fat milk, non-fat milk, natural juices, and bottled water. Ask that regular vending machines be filled with reduced-fat crackers, dried fruit, and low-fat cereal bars.

- Lobby for longer lunch periods. One reason a lot of teens get their lunch from vending machines is that the school lunch lines are so long that there's not enough time to eat. Eating a candy bar and chips from the vending machine saves you from starving. But with a longer lunch period, you won't be forced to grab food on the run.

- Tell the powers that be that you don't necessarily want all the unhealthy food revoked, but tell them *you want choices.*

As I close this key, let me just share a brief story with you. I was talking to a girl named Steffi who discovered the power of creating a no-fail environment. Steffi got pregnant when she was 16. The stresses and stigma of being a teenage mom came crushing down on her, and she ate her way up to a dangerously heavy 200 pounds. When Steffi returned to high school that fall, she was the fattest—and most picked on—girl in school. But the real wake-up call came not so much from the rejection, but from the shock that she could not fit into the classroom desks. The humiliation of trying to squeeze into a desk, then being forced to sit in the back of the class on a bench, was more than she could bear.

But the humiliation was a blessing in disguise. It gave her the kick in the butt she needed to change her life. Steffi went home, poured her heart out to her mom, and with her mom's help, cleared the entire kitchen of junk food and snacks, replacing the fattening food with whole grains, fruits, vegetables, and low-fat proteins. Steffi began to see that she could get control of her environment and create a healthier life for herself. By the time summer rolled around, she had trimmed herself down to 120 pounds.

When I was talking to Steffi about this, she told me this:

Viewing Options: ➡view all messages ➡view all messages ➡outline view

UNTITLED MESSAGE

Choosing not to buy fattening foods or have them at home made things so much better for me. With my mother's help, I avoided foods I used to binge on or couldn't resist. At first, it was hard because I was so emotionally upset over my life and school. But I hung in there, and it got easier. I was bothered less and less by the foods that gave me trouble. After a while, I just didn't miss them. I was to the point where I could not look at a bag of chocolate chip cookies and say no. So, I planned ahead and made sure that I wouldn't have to look at a bag of chocolate chip cookies. It was hard to get rid of those cookies, but in the long run it made reaching my goals *much* easier.

➡reply to this message ➡add to favorites ➡view all replies

You may not have the option of clearing all the foods out of your mother's cabinets as Steffi did, but you can make other significant changes in your environment if you just look around you and see where you have the power and the control.

Action Plan

Certain people, places, things, and feelings are cues, or trouble spots, to reach for a fattening snack or automatically stuff ourselves, even if we're not hungry. There are lots of these cues in your environment, and many are pretty loud and powerful. But they won't get to you if you make decisions and take action to deal with them. When you do this, you make it practically impossible to fail at healthy weight control.

- What are your toughest environmental cues?

My biggest, toughest cues: _____

- Do you need to avoid these things for a while or can you deal with them in another way?

- Think of three things you can do with your friends this weekend that don't involve food.

_____

_____

_____

_____

- Is there a food that you probably eat too much of—like a milkshake every day, or cookies every day after school, or a double cheeseburger for lunch?

A better substitute for that food: _____

- Try to add up the money you spent on fast food or snacks last week. What else could you buy with the same amount of money that isn't food?

Suppose your mom let you help her with the grocery list this week.

Three healthy foods you would put on the list:

_____

_____

_____

Three fattening foods you would not put on the list:

_____

_____

_____

Controlling the cues in your environment is one of the coolest and best moves you can make to get in shape. You don't have to worry about going on some dumb diet when you do this—because fattening foods are out of sight and therefore out of mind. Plus, you can still go out with your friends because you know how to plan, prepare, and not cave in.

Chapter 7

Key 4: Mastery Over Food and Impulse Eating

Why You Need This Key:

To get rid of bad habits—so that you get what you really want.

What do you do that you just hate yourself for doing but still can't make yourself stop? Maybe you curl up in front of the TV every night and eat your way through a super-sized bag of Doritos. Maybe you go to five fast food restaurants in a row—devouring two double Whoppers and a large fries at Burger King, throwing that up, then moving on to McDonald's for Chicken McNuggets, and a shake, then throwing that up, and heading for Baskin-Robbins, and so on and so on. By the end of your eating frenzy you've spent $50 or $60 in a couple of hours and hurt yourself in the process. Or maybe you stay home every weekend, hiding in your own little world, isolating yourself from your friends, and never doing anything fun anymore because you're too afraid that if you go out you'll end up at the pizza place, like you always do, pigging out on double cheese and pepperoni.

Eventually it feels as if the habits are in control of you instead of you being in control of the habits. Like smokers who stand outside in the freezing cold or the pouring rain just to smoke a cigarette, maybe you too are controlled by your habits. So do you ever wonder why you keep doing these things to yourself when you know in your head that they're hurting you? Do you ever ask yourself why you feel as if you just can't stop, no matter how much you want to?

We all have bad habits. They are these behaviors we repeat, even though they make no sense whatsoever and are physically and emotionally damaging. Well, there is a reason we keep doing them. It's the power of the *payoff*. A payoff is kind of like a reward. I know it's hard to believe that part of you likes these terrible behaviors, but if you think about it, it really makes sense. In fact, I wrote about this idea in my first book, *Life Strategies for Teens*. As I mentioned in that book, the power of the payoff and its ability to make you do something that you just flat-out hate yourself for doing is an absolute law of life—*people do what works*. So in some way, even if you don't realize it, that behavior you hate is working for you.

It sounds really intense, and in a way it is. But once you know about your payoffs, you can find healthier ways to get those same rewards. That's how you break the cycle of destructive behaviors. This key will show you how to take control of these habits—in some really different ways that you have never tried or even heard of before. Once you really understand what I am saying here and apply it, your life will begin to change the moment you turn this key.

The Power of Payoffs

On the surface, you probably tell yourself that you don't like certain aspects of your behavior. You don't like stuffing yourself all the time, or you don't like throwing up your food. You don't like going on and off a different diet every two weeks or subjecting your body to hunger strikes. You don't like your obsessions with food, dieting, and trying to be thin. But the truth is, deep down, maybe at an unconscious level, these behaviors are giving you something you really want. They're giving you a quick fix, an immediate reward. They're giving you a payoff.

I'm sure you're thinking, "Why in the world would I keep doing something I don't like? That doesn't make any sense." You're exactly right, it doesn't make any sense and I know it's hard to get your head around, but please hang in there with me on this one: The fact is, we repeat behaviors only if the results are satisfying in some way. For instance, think about why girls shave their legs (or guys their face). Is it fun? No. Do they enjoy it? No. It's a pain. And they wouldn't do it if it didn't give the payoff of smoother, more attractive legs (or face). So, that behavior works for them.

On the other hand, if you do something and get a crappy result, you're not going to do it again. It's not a very complicated concept. Here's the oldest example in the book: If a kid touches a hot stove and burns his hand, he learns not to touch it again, because it hurt. Imagine you teased the neighbor's Rottweiler and it bit you. Think you'll do that again? No way. You won't repeat the behavior because it did not work for you.

So far I haven't really said anything amazing, right? Basically, if you like the results of something you will do it again, and if you don't like the results, you won't. So, based on that, if you are repeating some behavior, you must like the result. The catch is that you may be saying "But that is the thing; I am repeating behaviors that lead to consequences I don't like." If that is the case, then you must like the results at some level, and in this chapter we are going to start identifying those things that you like, even though you may not realize it.

Are you with me so far? What I am saying is that if you are repeating food and eating-related behaviors that you consciously know are not good for you, then those behaviors must be working for you on a subconscious level, in ways you may not even be aware of. It doesn't matter if you know that overeating can lead to heart disease, diabetes, or cancer someday. It doesn't matter if you know that purposely throwing up your food can rupture your esophagus if you keep doing it. It doesn't matter that you are taking diet pills that can lead to heart problems, stroke, or kidney failure. It doesn't matter because somewhere deep down, the immediate payoff that comes from these behaviors is more important. Just because you're not conscious of the payoff, doesn't mean it's not there.

Now here's why all this information is important: If you want to stop your nasty habits once and for all—and instead manage your weight in a healthy way that actually works—then you have to find out what you're getting from these behaviors that makes you keep doing them. In other words, you have to figure out your payoffs. It's not good enough to say, "Oh, I wish I didn't eat so much," or "I wish I didn't puke after every meal," or "I wish I could stop gaining weight." You have to discover what is really going on inside that makes you act in such a self-destructive way when it comes to food, eating, and your body. If you can do that, you'll have a major tool to stop hurting and hating yourself, and start living a much better life.

I want to introduce you to a group of teens I sat down with recently who were brave enough to tell me about their bad food-related habits, which they hate doing, but just can't seem to stop. See if you can relate to their stories.

Viewing Options: ➡️ view all messages ➡️ view all messages ➡️ outline view

UNTITLED MESSAGE

My mom's a really good cook. I love all the stuff she makes, like mashed potatoes and homemade banana bread. It tastes so good. And yeah, I eat a lot of it. I don't really know why. It's just fun to eat, I guess, even though I know I'm about 20 pounds overweight. I should lose some weight, but I just like eating. I always have. Every bite that I put in my mouth I imagine sticking to my belly and instantly making me fatter. I look at a plate of food and I just see me getting bigger, but I still go back for seconds and dessert. I just can't stop!
—Jim, age 16

➡️ reply to this message ➡️ add to favorites ➡️ view all replies

Viewing Options: ➡ view all messages ➡ view all messages ➡ outline view

UNTITLED MESSAGE

My home is a very scary place to be. My dad's an alcoholic. When he's drinking, he gets violent. He slaps my mom around, and other times he hits my brother and me. I never know when he's going to come home drunk, or when the violence is going to break out. It's so chaotic and frightening that I just start eating and I can't stop. Then I feel guilty about all the weight I know I'm going to gain, so I throw up the food. I feel better after I get rid of the food, but only for a little while. Then I start to hate myself because I feel trapped in this cycle, like I have no control. But when the drinking, the yelling, and the fighting start, it's like, I automatically turn to food, and vomit it up later.

—Carrie, age 17

➡ reply to this message ➡ add to favorites ➡ view all replies

Viewing Options: ➡ view all messages ➡ view all messages ➡ outline view

UNTITLED MESSAGE

I weigh almost 200 pounds, which is way too heavy for my height. No guys ever ask me out, and in a way, I like that. Attention from guys makes me start to panic—it has ever since I was 9, when my older male cousin made me take all my clothes off and then molested me. A lot of times, though, I do feel really lonely and left out. So I try to go on a diet. For a while, I do pretty well and I lose a lot of weight. But as soon as a guy wants to ask me out, I get really anxious and freak out, and I just go back to bingeing on bowl after bowl of ice cream. It's the only thing that calms me down and makes me feel better, but I also gain back all the weight. I hate wasting

all of the progress that I have made (a.k.a. getting fat again), but it is almost as if getting fat again makes me happier than losing the weight and reaching my goal.
—Lisa, age 17

➡reply to this message ➡add to favorites ➡view all replies

Viewing Options: ➡view all messages ➡view all messages ➡outline view

UNTITLED MESSAGE

Some of the time, I eat pretty healthy, but I'm trying to lose weight because I'm 25 pounds bigger than I should be. Whenever I get good grades, or make an A on an assignment, I treat myself with cheeseburgers and fries—lots of them. I make really good grades all the time though, so the amount of food I'm eating is catching up with me. It seems like I'm getting bigger by the week. I hate the weight I've gained. But eating to celebrate good grades is something I just do. It doesn't feel the same if I don't. I like to eat, and that is one of the few rewards that I can give myself.
—Luke, age 15

➡reply to this message ➡add to favorites ➡view all replies

Viewing Options: ➡view all messages ➡view all messages ➡outline view

UNTITLED MESSAGE

My friends love to eat. We order pizza every time we sleep over at each other's houses and have donuts the next morning before we go home. We're always going out for ice cream. It just seems like everything we do revolves around food. I am worried about how I look, and I don't want to eat all that food because it always makes me feel really gross. But if I don't eat what they eat, or if I want do something else, they get mad at me. I don't know which is worse: eating so much junk food or feeling like a loser. Eating is just easier. I always tell myself that I will just work out twice as hard tomorrow, but I know that it doesn't work that way.

—Ashley, age 14

➡️reply to this message ➡️add to favorites ➡️view all replies

Viewing Options: ➡️view all messages ➡️view all messages ➡️outline view

UNTITLED MESSAGE

Last summer I went to fat camp—that's what everyone calls it. It's weight loss camp for teens. I lost 18 pounds and looked really good. Nobody could believe it. Everybody kept complimenting me on how great I looked. My mom bought me all new clothes for school. But then I started gaining a few pounds back. It really scared me. I got petrified that people wouldn't think I was cute anymore and that I'd let my mom down. So I became really strict and kept on dieting, to the point where now I hardly eat anything at all. I hate it. I am always hungry and constantly worried about calories, and fat, and carbs. It just gets really old!

—Marla, age 16

➡️reply to this message ➡️add to favorites ➡️view all replies

Does any of this sound familiar? Maybe you have some of these habits yourself or ones of your own that I didn't go over. Well, if you do, you now know it's because you need the payoff you get from those behaviors. Whether or not you can admit it right now, those payoffs are a huge factor in shaping how you act.

Let's get a little more specific about these payoffs. For Jim, the payoff from eating is as simple as pleasure. The enjoyment he gets from eating certain foods outweighs the satisfaction he'd get from being at a healthy weight. It's a natural tendency—most of us seek pleasure and avoid pain. But Jim's pleasure-seeking behavior is going to cause him a lot of problems down the road.

Carrie relies on her bulimia to deal with fear. Stuffing herself and then purging everything releases the tension and anxiety she feels when her dad gets violent. It calms and soothes her, it makes her feel in control, and that's her payoff.

Lisa keeps overeating because she finds some psychological comfort in food—and in her weight. She gets a payoff from staying fat. It's Lisa's way of making sure that guys won't ask her out. It's as if the fat is some kind of protective shield; when she's heavy she feels safe. She is scared of guys looking at her the way her cousin once did, and when she is fat, no guys look at her like that.

For Luke, pigging out every time he gets a good grade makes his success into more of a ceremony. It makes the occasion feel more special, like more of a big deal. That's his payoff. Even though he knows this behavior is making him fat, he justifies it as a reward for his hard work. But Luke's just kidding himself. Rewarding yourself with food every now and then is okay, but it becomes a problem when you do it all the time. There are other ways for Luke to reward himself that are healthier, but just as satisfying. When you start to "use" food for things other than nutrition it can really become a problem.

Ashley eats what the crowd eats because she needs acceptance. Even though she worries about gaining weight, for her, fitting in is even more important, so she caves in to the peer pressure.

With Marla, the payoff is the positive attention she receives. She doesn't feel good about herself without other people giving her the positive attention and compliments. So to keep it coming, she's always dieting. The problem is, she's going to extreme measures to stay thin, and now she's on the verge of anorexia.

There is nothing wrong with enjoying food, relieving tension, needing comfort, wanting to belong, rewarding yourself, seeking immediate gratification, or liking compliments. The payoffs we get are not really the harmful part. It's the self-destructive and self-defeating behaviors we use to get to the payoffs that are the problem. But luckily, a payoff is a payoff no matter where it comes from, and there are better, healthier ways to get the same results. I want you to have the payoffs, just without the dangerous habits.

To find healthy behaviors that will get you the same rewards, the first thing you have to do is identify bad behaviors and the payoffs they bring. Look at this chart and see if you find yourself in here some way.

Negative Behavior	Payoffs
Overeating	Distraction from stress; comfort and calm; weight gain to keep unattractive to the opposite sex; protection/safety from rejection; unhealthy reward system
Going on and off diets	Attention; peer pressure; acceptance
Eating too much junk food	Instant satisfaction; peer acceptance; unhealthy reward system; convenience
Mindless snacking	Distraction from stress
Bingeing	Numb negative emotions; tension release; anger or rebellion
Purging	Emotional relief; cleansing (allows you to get rid of "dirtiness" inside you)

Starving	Protection/safety of a small body; control in a world run by others; attention
Using diet pills	Need for a quick fix

Finding Your Payoffs

Let's talk more about why you do things you don't want to do. In the space below, or in your journal, take some time to list at least five of the most frustrating self-destructive behaviors in your life—behaviors that relate to food, eating, dieting, or your weight. They have to be behaviors that are bad for you. Answer this question: "What are you doing with food, eating, or your body that you would like to stop?" Write down what you do that makes you say "I hate myself for doing that."

1. _____
2. _____
3. _____
4. _____
5. _____

Now, in the space below, or in your journal, write down what you think the payoff, or payoffs, are for each of these behaviors. To help figure this out, think about when you use these behaviors, and what you are feeling when you do. You might have to dig deep, but this exercise will be worth the effort. When you understand what your payoffs are, you can make more thoughtful, healthier choices in your life.

1. _____
2. _____
3. _____
4. _____
5. _____

Action Steps

By writing down the info in the previous exercise you've just taken a huge step toward making positive changes—acknowledging that you're unhappy with the way things are and identifying the payoffs that drive your actions. But to get better results, you have to choose better behaviors. That's where we're headed next.

Step 1: Replace Bad Habits With Incompatible Actions

A bad habit can be a stubborn thing, but it is completely possible to break it. You just have to replace your bad habit with healthy behavior. And that new behavior has to be *incompatible* with the old one. Whatever the new behavior is, it cannot coexist with overeating, bingeing, purging, or any other self-destructive behavior. For example, it's pretty hard to plow through a bag of Hershey's Kisses if you're taking a shower; because taking a shower is incompatible with inhaling chocolate Kisses.

There are plenty of others: It's difficult to do your workout video while eating a big bucket of KFC. Eating fried chicken is incompatible with working out. It's tough to throw up if you're sitting at your desk writing down your feelings in your journal. Vomiting is incompatible with journal writing.

Okay, I know you get it—no more examples. But finding a behavior that interferes with the one you want to ditch is a good way to eliminate that habit. Why? First of all, like we said, doing the healthy one does not allow you to do the unhealthy one. But second, it also takes your mind off the habit you want to lose. If you're focusing on doing something positive, there's no room for your brain to think about the negative.

What I'm asking you to do is probably the opposite of what you're used to. You are probably really good at "multitasking." You can do a million different things at once—like talking on the phone, checking your e-mail, and doing your homework, all while wearing your Crest Whitestrips. But that's not what you want to do when you're working on changing a habit. Instead, focus on the substitution of the bad habit with a healthier one.

Okay, let's make this discussion practical by listing some of the activities you can use to stop overeating, bingeing, purging, or any other weight- and body-sabotaging behaviors (because they're incompatible).

To help you think through this, here are some ideas, organized into three broad categories: fun stuff or things you do because you enjoy them; relaxation activities or things you can do to relieve stress and tension; and must-do's or obligations you have to your parents or to your schoolwork.

Fun

- Shoot hoops.

- Dance or sing to some upbeat music.

- Play some games on your Xbox.

- Throw a Frisbee around.

- Play some Free Cell on your computer.

- Give yourself a manicure or pedicure.

- Pursue a favorite hobby, like photography or painting.

- Play the guitar or another musical instrument.

- Take a walk.

- Throw the football around.

- Do push-ups or sit-ups.

- Go to a friend's house.

- Go clothes shopping.

Relaxation

- Breathe (deep breathing as a way to relax and get focused).

- Go running.

- Lift weights at the gym.

- Hit a punching bag or a pillow.

- Write in your journal.

- Sing.

- Take a shower or bubble bath.

- Pamper yourself with a facial.

- Take a walk.

- Take a short nap.

- Write a poem or compose a song.

- Pray or meditate.

Must-Do's

- Do your homework.

- Finish your chores around the house.

- Clean your room.

- Run errands for your mother.

- Practice a musical instrument.

- Walk your dog.

- Do all the things your dentist keeps telling you to do: brush, floss, rinse with mouthwash.

- Volunteer: Serve food at a shelter or have your long hair chopped off for a good cause.

- Reach out to someone who needs help.

Now I want you to add to the list. Come up with specific activities that have nothing to do with food that you can personally use as alternatives. There are two requirements: The activities you select must be available at a moment's notice, and they must be incompatible with the habit you're trying to break.

Short of tattooing the list on your body (don't), do everything you can to always have this list handy. Put it in your purse, tape it to the mirror in your bedroom, keep it in the glove compartment of your car, save it on your computer, write it in your notebooks, and hang it in your locker. As soon as you feel like doing your bad habit, ask yourself, "What can I do instead?" Look at your list and immediately do one of these incompatible activities. In a really short amount of time, you'll begin to conquer the bad behavior.

Step 2: Stop Your Impulses and Urges

Young people are short on what psychologists like to call "impulse control." That's why you yell, "I hate you!" at your mom one minute and are laughing with her the next, or why you do seriously stupid things like getting in a car with someone who's driving drunk. It's also why you so easily inhale an entire bag of Sun Chips without thinking about it.

Part of the reason for this is that our brain is a work in progress. From our teens into our twenties, the parts of our brain responsible for judgment, self-control, regulation of emotions, and insight are still developing. Because they haven't fully matured, we're easily distracted, little things make us nuts, and we're impulsive.

To make matters worse, the cues we talked about in the previous key—thoughts and feelings, the sight and smell of food, people or places—can weaken whatever impulse control you do have, so you tend to give in to urges more easily. These urges are called "impulse moments," and you can expect to experience four to seven of them a day.

In order to successfully manage your weight, you have to learn how to deal with these impulse moments when they hit. Otherwise you'll default to your self-destructive behavior. The first thing to do is figure out when impulse moments are most likely to nail you. Is it a certain time of day? When you get home from school and you're alone in the house? Or when you're plopped on the couch watching TV? Do you feel the urge to splurge when you're tired?

Once you figure out where and when you're most vulnerable, you can deliberately use a new incompatible behavior from your list. The substitute activity will help you switch gears, so you'll stop thinking about food, eating, or weight. You will change your entire way of coping. Sure this requires a little bit of energy and thought, but trust me, if you do this, the impulse moments will pass as quickly as they hit. Just keep practicing. Don't give up. Old habits die hard, but they do die.

Step 3: Change Your Eating Style

There are other behaviors that will trip you up, big-time. They have to do with how you interact with food. I call them fast eating, whole-thing eating, and grab-and-go eating.

Fast Eating

I once did an experiment. I sat in a fast food restaurant and observed a lot of rather large people eat, teens included. (I made sure nobody could tell I was watching.) All these people had one thing in common. They ate their food faster than a malnourished *Survivor* contestant just voted off the island. Their mouths were full of food at all times, and they held their burgers hovering near their lips so the food was ready for another bite as soon as they swallowed. No one talked much; some of them didn't even look up. They just ate . . . and ate . . . and ate. I got full just watching them.

What I saw wasn't unusual: On average, people who are overweight eat faster than ones who aren't, according to obesity experts. Even though taste is a powerful cue for eating, overweight people eat too fast to even taste their food. This eating behavior—gulping down food very rapidly—is part of the reason they pack on pounds. Fast eating defeats the messages your brain sends out that say "Stop eating, you're full." So you keep on eating, past the point of necessity.

If you eat more slowly, you can better control how much food you eat overall. When you eat slowly, you need less food to feel satisfied. It's really simple but it's a great trick for weight management. Here are some other ways to put the brakes on your fast eating:

- Wait five minutes before you eat the food that's placed in front of you.

- Put small amounts of food on your fork or spoon.

- Use smaller utensils (try a cocktail fork, for example)—no soup spoons, ladles, or otherwise oversized tableware for shoveling in food.

- Put your utensils down between every bite.

- Consciously take time to taste and chew—savor your food.

- Completely swallow food from each mouthful before you add any more to your fork or spoon.

- Take sips of water or other noncaloric beverages between bites.

Just eating more slowly will cause you to eat less and thus lose weight. Give it a shot because this tip is really easy to do.

Whole-Thing Eating

It's like a law of physics or something: The more food that's on your plate, the more you eat. If you super-sized your meal, or pile too much food on your plate at once, you'll probably eat the whole thing. The bigger the portions, the more we put away.

As you learned in the previous key, extra-large servings at "value" prices are a marketing ploy to get you to buy—and as a result eat—more than you need. But if you care about healthy weight management, you have to find a way to deal with it. Here are some strategies:

- When you eat out with a friend, order one meal and ask for two plates so that you can split it.

- At restaurants, eat only half your meal, then get the rest to go (cut everything in half before you ever take a bite).

- Stop super-sizing it; go for regular or kiddie portions instead.

- Just say no to seconds.

Grab-and-Go Eating

Teens are busy. You're caught up in the daily rush of school, homework, extracurricular activities, after-school jobs, and time with your friends. Many of you also have to fend for yourself when it comes to meals, because you live with a single parent, or both of your parents work. It's no wonder your eating habits are so crazy. With no set times for breakfast, lunch, or dinner, you just *grab* and *go*.

Unfortunately, this eating pattern is another reason for unhealthy weight gain. When you have a few minutes to just eat whatever's convenient, you tend to choose less nutritious foods and give in to cravings. If you don't know how to stop grab-and-go eating, I've got some suggestions listed below. They'll help you get this aspect of your eating behavior under better control.

- Plan when you're going to eat. Pick regular time slots for your three meals and two snacks a day. If it helps, write down what you'll eat in advance. Taking the time to figure out a schedule, and then writing it down, gives you a greater sense of control.

- Get in the habit of eating breakfast. If you don't use any of the other tips, at least do this one. Teens and children who do pay more attention in school, can solve more complex problems in math, science, and other subjects, and get better grades.

- "Localize" your eating. Select one table in your house—in the dining room, breakfast nook, or some other area reserved only for eating—and eat *all* of your food there. At school, eat only in the cafeteria.

- If you're going to eat, don't do anything else. Don't eat while you're driving; or standing in front of the open refrigerator, or even reading a book or magazine, sitting in your bed, or talking on the phone. Doing so distracts your attention from your eating behavior, and you'll lose all awareness of how much food you're actually eating.

Step 4: Stop Your Dieting Behavior

I am seriously anti-diet. Dieting is as much a behavior as eating, overeating, bingeing, purging, exercising, or not exercising. Repeatedly going on and off diets all the time is one of the most self-destructive and frustrating behavior patterns you can have.

Diets have been the downfall for way too many teens. That's because dieting is actually one of the main behaviors that leads to weight problems and eating disorders, according to the psychologists and nutritionists I worked with. Most people who go on a diet regain the weight they lose, plus more, within a few years. People who become bulimic or anorexic almost always started down that road with a diet. Dieting can result in a sick preoccupation with food and with your body and weight, which is just plain unhealthy. When dieting fails—and it almost always does—people may resort to purging or starving to control their weight. So when you decide to "go on a diet," you are setting yourself up for failure, because you may never get the results you want. Diets just don't work. Look at it this way: If dieting worked, you'd only have to do it once.

The payoff of a diet is the feeling that you have control over your weight. But it's a false sense of control. Think about it: Is it really control if you regain all the weight as soon as you go off the diet?

This advice to skip dieting is even more important for teens than it is for adults. Why? Because your body is growing and developing right now—you're in transition—and being on some idiotic diet at this stage in your life can be unhealthy and interfere with your growth. Dieting is not cool. It's self-destructive.

Make a deal with me: While you are learning these keys and putting them into action, you will not go on a diet. Say good-bye to that behavior, at least for as long as you're reading this book. Instead, work on making healthy choices by following the seven keys. Take positive steps. Lose the diets.

Healthy Payoffs From Healthy Behaviors

Let's wind up the same way we started—by talking about payoffs. Most of the new, incompatible activities we've come up with here will generate the same payoffs you used to get from overeating, bingeing, starving yourself, and all those other negative behaviors. Exercise is a good example. Exercising, whether it involves going to the gym or walking around the block a few times, produces the same high you get from food. So do relaxation, meditation, or listening to music. Even cleaning your room or doing your homework can give you a sense of accomplishment, while taking your mind off food. Simple behaviors like eating slowly, controlling your portions, and having breakfast produce payoffs like good grades and feeling and looking great.

Just about every constructive activity you can substitute for negative eating behaviors can generate the payoffs you want, but in a much healthier way. As my dad always says, "When you choose the behavior, you choose the consequences." If you use this key, you will choose the consequences of getting in much better shape.

Action Plan

If you are overeating, bingeing, purging, or doing something else you don't like, you are doing it for a reason—for the payoff it gives you. The first step toward stopping this stuff is figuring out your payoffs. Once you do that, you can start replacing a bad habit with an incompatible substitute—something that gives you the same payoff but in a healthier way.

- What is the most powerful payoff you're getting from the behavior you want to stop? What do you get from this behavior or habit? What are some other ways to get the same payoff, but without the negative consequence?

- Ask yourself which of the bad food or eating habits, or other self-destructive behaviors discussed in this key, do you have the most trouble with.

The eating or food habit that I struggle most with:

_____

- Make it your goal to go through one week without doing it. (Use your list of incompatible substitutes to help you.)

My plan for dealing with this habit(s):

_____
_____
_____
_____
_____

Sure, bad habits are a bummer. But when you use these action steps and make a plan, you get in control of your habits. Your bad habits are not in control of you.

Chapter 8

Key 5: Jay's Portion Power Plan

Why You Need This Key:

To look good and feel great by making the right nutritional choices.

D o you ever wish you could get in shape without another crazy diet? Wouldn't it be nice if you could get your eating under control, and not be so preoccupied with food? Do you want to enjoy food without worrying about gaining weight? If so, you're going to love Key 5 because it is the solution to these problems.

Key 5 is all about learning a better way to eat, one that helps you look your best, do your best, and be your best. It is about choosing foods that work for you, and limiting those that don't. It is a way to break bad eating patterns.

Over the next several pages, we'll go through the nutritional steps necessary to do this—and more. But first, I have something important to tell you: Some of why you're overweight, or in the grip of an eating disorder, is not entirely your fault. It really isn't. I don't want you to blame others. I just want you to realize that you have been influenced to eat the way you do by a lot of different forces out there. We are going to go over those now.

Family and School Forces

Pretend that I'm whispering this to you so your parents and teachers won't hear: You've grown up with bad nutrition, and now that's all you know. A lot of what you've been taught at home and at school is misleading, incorrect, and making you fat or, in a lot of cases, obsessed with dieting and getting thin.

When you were little, you depended on your parents or other

adults to make choices for you. Questions about what to eat, for example, were probably all answered with little or no input from you, but by the adults in your life, usually genuinely thinking they were acting in your best interests. Your mom, dad, and grandparents may have used food as a reward or punishment. When you were good, they may have rewarded you with cookies and candy, or they punished you with no dessert when you drew all over the living room wall with your crayons. You may have gotten into the habit of "cleaning your plate" because your parents told you to. Or maybe they forbade junk food to the point that that's all you could think about, so you started to sneak it at friends' houses. Your parents also *modeled* (set an example of) what to eat and what not to eat, and you followed them. You ate the way they ate. If they ate a lot of food high in fat, sugar, and calories, then you learned to do the same, and now maybe it has become habit, or even addictive. You did this innocently, without knowing the consequences of your choices. Those consequences include being overweight or susceptible to eating disorders, and associated problems like feeling depressed, stuck, or a little psycho at times.

When you got to school, your teachers taught you the food guide pyramid, but that nutrition tool is undergoing a much-needed revision. It tells you to eat six to eleven servings of carbohydrates, which is way too much. It doesn't differentiate between natural carbs (like whole grains) and processed carbs like cookies. Putting away that many carbs every day could take you all the way to plus-size elastic pants.

I'm not talking about blaming your parents or your schools. But if you're going to get real about your problems with weight and food, you've got to recognize how much you carry with you from these childhood models, even if you don't realize it. You've been programmed like a computer, but you may have been programmed with bad information.

America's Other "Drug" Problem

Meet Angie, who's 17. At this moment, she's having a craving so overwhelming that she has no choice but to satisfy it. She is desperately tearing through the house looking for her fix. Nothing else matters. Angie raids the kitchen, looking everywhere for something chocolate. She can't find anything and starts to get desperate. She digs for lint-covered change at the bottom of her backpack and searches her mom's purse for loose dollar bills. Then she drives to the nearest convenience store. She walks in and buys a fistful of candy bars, making some excuse about buying for her friends—she's embarrassed about how many candy bars she's about to eat by herself, but that doesn't stop her. Once she gets to the car, she stuffs them in her mouth fast. She feels a physical and mental high that will last for an hour or two.

Angie is an addict, and her drug is sugar. She knows all about the dangers of getting drunk, smoking, snorting, and shooting up, but what she doesn't know are the dangers of overeating sugar—the number-one food additive.

Sugar? A drug? How is that possible?

Psychologists and eating disorder specialists say that the taste of sugar may excite the same wiring in your brain that is stimulated by pleasure-inducing drugs. It delivers a mild and short-lived high. Foods that contain added sugar—along with fat and salt—can be, for many people, as addictive as cigarettes, drugs, or alcohol. They can be just as difficult to give up. They carry with them terrible side effects such as weight gain and the problems that go along with it.

Sugar consumption is out of control. On average, if you're a teenage guy, you eat at least 109 pounds of sugar a year—probably almost as much as your girlfriend weighs. A lot of this is in the form of sugary soft drinks, which are basically "liquid candy." Teens as a whole are drinking roughly 160 gallons of soft drinks a year—which breaks down to about 2 quarts a day. It's actually kind of nauseating when you think about it that way! Experts place a lot of the blame for teenage obesity on this single food behavior.

A lot of what you're eating has been purposely concocted with sugar, fat, and salt to hook you, without your even knowing it. But the good news is that you can detox from this junk. It can be hard at first. But once sugar and the processed carbs that contain it are out of your body, and you eat moderate and regularly scheduled meals, it gets easier because the physical cravings go away.

Portion Distortion

It's not only what we eat, but also how much we eat that's important. The portion sizes at restaurants are getting bigger and bigger. Many restaurant meals supply a half day's worth of calories! Even a "small" bucket of popcorn at the movie theater holds 7 cups of popcorn and 400 calories. Go to any fast food restaurant and on the menu you will find not only large, medium, and small, but "king-sized," "queen-sized," "monster meals," and "biggie" items. There's even a word in your vocabulary to describe this— "super-size"—courtesy of McDonald's. It may sound like a good deal when you are ordering, but think about this: If you super-size your meals, you may super-size your body—and your problems with food.

Fast Food Mania

Speaking of fast food: It's everywhere! On billboards, on TV, and in magazines, they're pushing fast food to millions of consumers—teens included—only too willing to eat them up. Burger King alone sells 4 million Whoppers a day!

A typical fast food meal (double cheeseburger, French fries, a soft drink, and a dessert) weighs in at about 2,200 calories—that is a whole day's worth of calories. One report I read found that teenage girls who eat out at fast food restaurants several times a week take in roughly 260 extra, unneeded calories each time. That equates to a 15-pound weight gain in one year! And to make matters worse, they do everything to get us hooked. Think about it: When we were kids, they would give us toys if we would eat their fast food.

I'm not knocking fast food. There are actually a lot of choices you can make at fast food restaurants that are pretty healthy, and we'll be talking about them in this key.

To sum up: You've been unknowingly programmed to eat a lot of crap that's not good for you, and now things may be out of control. That is not to say you can't change—you can. The past is past, and this is a new beginning. This is a time of your life when you are breaking away from your family and becoming more and more independent. You're learning how to make choices for yourself—and those choices include what to eat and drink. Getting healthy and feeling great are about making choices that help your body operate at its very best.

Food Choice Quiz

What about you? Are your food choices healthy or harmful? Take this quick quiz to find out. Circle the answer that describes what you do most of the time.

1. **Which of these meals do you usually eat on the weekends?**
   a. Lean meat and salad, lots of veggies.
   b. Pizza, usually with a side salad or vegetable.
   c. Burgers, cheeseburgers, tacos, pizza, or other fast food.

2. **For sandwiches, which type of bread do you usually eat?**
   a. Whole wheat.
   b. Sometimes whole wheat, sometimes white bread.
   c. White bread, mostly.

3. **Complete this sentence: When I go to a fast food restaurant,**
   a. I don't eat fast foods that much.
   b. I usually order normal-sized portions of burgers and fries.
   c. I usually order the biggest portions on the menu.

4. **Which of these snacks are you most likely to munch on?**
   a. Fresh fruit or vegetables.
   b. Sometimes chips or sweets, sometime fruits or vegetables.
   c. Chips or sweets.

5. Which of these lunches do you typically eat at the school cafeteria?
   a. I pack my own lunch.
   b. I try to choose what looks healthy, if it's on the menu.
   c. Burgers and fries or chips.

6. When you get thirsty, what do you usually drink?
   a. Water
   b. Juice or juice drinks
   c. Soft drinks (regular)

7. When you want something sweet, what do you usually choose?
   a. Dried or fresh fruit.
   b. Some type of low-fat dessert or low-fat ice cream.
   c. Candy, popsicles, pastries, cookies, or other baked sweet.

8. Which of these breakfasts are you mostly likely to eat?
   a. Cereal, milk, and fresh fruit.
   b. Pancakes and sausage, or eggs and bacon.
   c. I usually skip breakfast.

9. On average, how often do you drink milk, or eat yogurt or cheese?
   a. Two to three times a day.
   b. Several times a week.
   c. Hardly ever.

10. How often do you diet?
   a. I don't diet. I try to eat healthy and to exercise.
   b. I go on a diet whenever I need to lose a few pounds.
   c. I'm always on some kind of new diet.

Scoring

Give yourself 2 points for each *a* answer; 1 point for each *b* answer; and 0 points for each *c* answer. Add up your score. If you scored 15 to 20, you make nutrition-smart choices. Keep up the good work. If you scored 6 to 14, your nutritional habits have room for improvement. If you scored 0 to 5, you need to change a lot about the way you're eating. Pay close attention to the steps in this key.

Making Food Choices

Okay, if your nutrition needs some polishing up, or if you want to increase your energy and improve your appearance, what should you eat?

Right now is the time in the book where I get to give you my take on what foods are best to choose for peak physical and mental performance. This information is based on what I learned from working with a nutritionist. This is not rocket science, either, just plain common sense on what's good for your body.

Power Proteins

This category of foods furnishes protein, a nutrient that gives your muscles size and shape and makes your body firm. Examples include lean meats, fish, poultry, and eggs. If you're following a good vegetarian diet, you can choose protein substitutes like beans, rather than animal-based ones. For healthy weight management, it's smart to have a food from this category at every meal, since protein is filling and keeps you from overeating.

Lean Dairy Foods

These foods provide calcium and other bone-building nutrients. One of these nutrients is vitamin D. You get it from drinking
milk and being out in the sun. But here's the catch: A lot of teens
don't drink milk, opting instead for soft drinks. They don't go outside much, either, because they're too busy on the Internet or
watching TV.

What's happening is that you're not getting enough vitamin D.
That's bad. It can stunt your growth and make your bones weak.
So you need to make sure you're eating enough dairy products
each day. Good choices in this category include low-fat milk, skim
milk, yogurt, cottage cheese, reduced-fat cheese, and low-fat,
sugar-free ice cream.

Fit Fruits

Fruits are loaded with nutrient all-stars like vitamins and minerals that make your skin glow and help your body run at its best.
This category includes fresh fruits, 100 percent fruit juice, and
fruits canned without added sugar.

Non-Starchy Vegetables

These foods supply a lot of vitamins, minerals, fiber (good
for healthy digestion and helping you feel full), and other health-
building nutrients. They include fresh and cooked vegetables such
as salad vegetables, green beans, cauliflower, lettuce, and tomatoes. Veggies do a lot for your skin, your energy level, and everything about how you feel.

Natural Carbs

These foods are high in energy-giving carbohydrates, which fuel your body and your brain for good physical and mental performance. Examples of these foods include whole-grain breads such as wheat bread; whole-grain cereals like oatmeal; whole-grain pastas; and starchy vegetables like potatoes, yams, and kidney beans.

Healthy Fats

Fats get a pretty bad rap, but some are very good for you. For example: olive oil, canola oil, flaxseed oil, other vegetable oils, nuts and seeds, reduced-fat peanut butter, and reduced-fat salad dressings.

You probably noticed that the following foods didn't make the list: candy, cake, cookies, donuts, pastries, high-fat lunch meats, sugary sodas and soft drinks, and snack foods such as crackers, potato chips, tortilla chips, corn chips, and cheese curls. These foods all taste great and are fun to eat. And some of them live up to their reputation as "comfort foods." For example, carbs like cookies, cakes, and pastries actually calm short-term stress by curbing stress chemicals in your body when you're tense, according to some late-breaking nutritional info.

So I'm not calling for the mass extinction of these foods in your diet. But don't take it too far. Try to limit these foods to an occasional treat, if you can handle them without overeating them. But keep in mind that eating high-sugar, high-fat foods as a habit will pack on unwanted, ugly pounds.

Bottom line: Choose foods that work for you, not against you.

There is an expanded list of these foods (Supplement B) in the back of the book.

Now it's time to get to the heart of my nutritional plan.

Action Steps

One big reason why so many teens are overweight, and others have issues with food has to with portion size. The over-sized portions we see and get at restaurants have completely skewed our perceptions of what to eat at home and elsewhere. We think mega sizes are normal sizes!

My Portion Power Plan solves this problem by giving you some portion-control techniques to downsize your body, your portions, and your problems with food. You'll learn to judge for yourself how much you really need to eat. This plan also keeps your hunger in check and curbs your craving for junk food. It accounts for the often crazy eating patterns we have, but at the same time, helps you reestablish regular meal patterns—which is important if your eating is out of control. Once you put this plan into action, you'll begin to look and feel better, starting almost right away.

Step 1: Exercise Your Portion Power

Portion power means supplying your body with exactly what it needs to be healthy and in shape—no more, no less. Every book I've ever seen tells us to eat 4 ounces of this or 7 ounces of that. Well, I have no idea how much 7 ounces is, and I refuse to carry a freaking scale everywhere.

To help you figure out how much the average teen should try to eat each day, I've developed a system of portions to illustrate exactly what your serving sizes should look like, relative to everyday items, including your own hand. It gives you a way to easily judge your portion sizes, at restaurants and at home (without having to mess with measuring cups or food scales), so that you won't be vulnerable to super-sizing. This chart shows how I've translated acceptable conventional portions into sizes you can easily recognize. (Of course, if you have any special dietary requirements or health problems, you should check with a doctor or nutritionist about recommended foods and portion size.)

Food	Jay's Portions	Conventional Portions
Power proteins like meat, fish, or poultry; or meat alternates like beans	Computer mouse	3 to 4 ounces
Lean dairy foods like milk or yogurt	Your fist	1 cup
Fit fruits	Tennis ball	1 medium piece of fruit
Non-starchy vegetables	Baseball	1 cup
Natural carbs like rice, pasta, cereal, or starchy vegetables	Your cupped hand	½ cup
Healthy fats like oil, reduced-fat peanut butter, or salad dressing	Tip of your thumb to the first joint, or a regular spoon	1 teaspoon for regular fats; 2 teaspoons for reduced-fat versions
Bread or sandwich; cheese	Computer disk	1 slice

All you need to do is try to eat three servings from each of the six food groups. That's a total of 18 portions of different foods daily, spread over breakfast, lunch, and dinner, plus two or three snacks. This plan relieves you of having to count calories because the calories are already counted for you.

Oh, by the way, don't be afraid of calories. They're just a way to compute how much energy a food gives you after you eat it. You need hundreds of calories every day just to keep your heart pumping blood and your lungs breathing air. The exact number you need each day depends on whether you're a guy or a girl, and how active you are. For a guy who's athletic, the right amount of calories is around 2,800. But a girl who spends most of her time sitting around needs only around 1,600, and that's just to maintain her weight. To lose weight, most teens can do it with around 1,200 to 1,500 calories a day. Then when you've lost weight and want to keep it off, you can do that with about 2,200 calories, as long as you exercise your body at least several times a week. Like I said though, you don't have to fuss with calorie counting with my plan.

So when you need more food later on, either to maintain your weight or fuel yourself for exercise, you can add more portions, particularly from fruits, vegetables, and natural carbs. This is a flexible way to approach nutrition and healthy weight management. Plus, it's used by therapists to help people with eating disorders normalize their eating and structure their meals.

Step 2: Track Your Meals

During the time you are learning better nutritional habits, it helps to track your meals to see how well you're doing. You can do this by using the Portion Power Meal Tracker shown here. Each day, all you have to do is check off the servings you ate. (Don't worry if you don't always make the 18. Just do your best.)

Checking off what you eat is beneficial for a number of reasons:

- It builds better nutritional habits.

- It makes you more aware of your food behavior.

- It identifies places where you might not be getting enough of a certain food category.

- It shows you all the positive changes you're making from week to week.

So here it is. Really write down your progress.

Portion Power Meal Tracker						
Day	Power Proteins	Lean Dairy Foods	Fit Fruits	Non-Starchy Vegetables*	Natural Carbs	Healthy Fats
Sunday	☐☐☐	☐☐☐	☐☐☐	☐☐☐	☐☐☐	☐☐☐
Monday	☐☐☐	☐☐☐	☐☐☐	☐☐☐	☐☐☐	☐☐☐
Tuesday	☐☐☐	☐☐☐	☐☐☐	☐☐☐	☐☐☐	☐☐☐
Wednesday	☐☐☐	☐☐☐	☐☐☐	☐☐☐	☐☐☐	☐☐☐
Thursday	☐☐☐	☐☐☐	☐☐☐	☐☐☐	☐☐☐	☐☐☐
Friday	☐☐☐	☐☐☐	☐☐☐	☐☐☐	☐☐☐	☐☐☐
Saturday	☐☐☐	☐☐☐	☐☐☐	☐☐☐	☐☐☐	☐☐☐

* It's okay to eat *more* than three of these food groups each day. Three servings is the *minimum* requirement.

Step 3: Choose Foods That Control Your Hunger and Improve Your Eating Habits

Foods that control hunger? Improve eating habits? How is that possible?

True fact: There are foods that can help slow down your eating and keep hunger and food cravings in check. When you're planning and tracking your meals, using the guidelines above, you'll want to avoid *Gulp-and-Gain Foods* and choose mostly *Get-Full-and-Fit Foods*. Let me explain.

Gulp-and-Gain Foods

There are quite a few foods that encourage fast eating, a habit that leads to weight gain. A candy bar is a classic example. It's easy to grab, straight from a vending machine or near the register at a convenience store. Once in your mouth, it melts right there—barely any chewing required. It goes down fast, before your body's hunger signals kick in. It's high in sugar, and this leads to cravings for more sugar—and more candy bars. What happens is that you end up packing away much more food, calories, sugar, and fat than you need and a whole lot more than you really wanted. That's why I call these foods Gulp-and-Gain Foods.

Other examples of Gulp-and-Gain foods include candy; chocolate; puddings; chips; cookies; cake; brownies; donuts and pastries; ice cream and frozen desserts; soft drinks (with sugar); any high-calorie convenience food; foods that require very little chewing: shakes; certain fast foods like burritos and cheeseburgers; foods you grab and eat on the run, like toaster pastries; foods eaten directly from their packages, like snack cakes; easy-to-prepare processed foods, like microwavable burritos; and any food you'd call "junk food."

So what's my point? Eat fewer Gulp-and-Gain Foods. This will make a real difference in your eating habits, help you stop fast eating, and curb your hunger. Trying to change unwanted behavior is hard enough. You certainly don't want to make it even harder by eating foods that invite the exact behavior you want to stop!

Get-Full-and-Fit Foods

From the six categories of food in my Portion Power Plan, there are a lot of foods that take effort to chew and are filling. I call them Get-Full-and-Fit Foods. Examples are fresh fruits, raw vegetables, leafy green salads, soups, whole grains, and proteins like meat, poultry, or fish.

Why is this important?

You can't just inhale these foods. They take time to fix and chew; plus, they make you feel full afterwards. A lot of them contain fiber, a nutrient that prevents hunger by making you feel full. Your brain gets the message that your body is satisfied. You feel full, but you haven't stuffed yourself.

Bottom line: These foods help slow down your eating for better weight management and to defeat out-of-control eating. The more of these foods you include in your meals, the better your nutrition—and the better your food habits. (There is a huge long list of these foods in Supplement B, so check it out.)

Step 4: Make Your Snack Attack a Healthy One

Many of you are like me. When you're out with your friends, those get-togethers almost always involve snacking. Guys eat an average of ten snacks a week; girls eat even more—twelve snacks a week, according to a report I looked at on teenagers' nutritional habits. There's absolutely nothing wrong with snacking. It's fun, and it's a great way to fill in the nutritional blanks teens have in their lives—provided you fill in those blanks with *mostly* healthy snacks. Okay, I detect a chorus of loud yawns, but stay with me through this and I'll make a believer out of you.

Unhealthy snack choices—foods loaded with calories, fat, and added sugar—can have huge influences on us. If you don't think so, look at this chart, and check out the number of pounds you can pack on with poor snacking habits.

Snack Habits	Weekly Calorie Cost	Calorie Cost Per Year	Potential Weight Gain Per Year
Eating a chocolate candy bar every day instead of an apple	896 extra calories a week	46,600 extra calories a year	13 pounds
Drinking one regular soda a day, rather than having a calorie-free soda (or other no-cal drink)	1,008 extra calories a week	52,400 extra calories a year	15 pounds
Drinking a milk-shake five times a week, rather than a fruit smoothie (low-fat milk blended with fresh strawberries)	1,050 extra calories a week	54,600 extra calories a year	16 pounds
Eating a bowl of regular ice cream (280 calories) five times a week, rather than having a bowl of non-fat frozen yogurt instead (160 calories)	600 extra calories a week	31,200 extra calories a year	9 pounds

Snacking while watching television, five hours a week (136 extra calories per snack)	680 extra calories a week	35,360 extra calories a year	10 pounds
Snacking on a small popcorn at the movies, twice a week (400 calories)	800 extra calories a week	41,600 calories a year	12 pounds

I rest my case. You could be choosing too many snacks that can practically guarantee weight gain, plus hurt your health. But you can also stop doing that and start looking better and feeling better, right now. If you're serious about getting on track, you'll get serious about snacking for success.

Maybe you would like to make better snack choices, but you aren't sure what those choices are. Here are some practical suggestions for nutritious snacks that taste good and will help you establish better snacking habits.

Snacking for Success

Refreshers
Low-fat milk, skim milk, 100% fruit juice, vegetable juices, diet sodas, water

Munchies
Plain, low-fat, or air-popped popcorn; raw, cut-up veggies and dip (dip mix made with plain yogurt or non-fat sour cream); low-fat or reduced-fat crackers with low-fat cheese; flavored rice cakes

Fuelers

Protein shakes, fortified nutrition bars; low-fat granola bars

Coolers

Low-fat ice milk, frozen yogurt, or pudding; sorbet; sugar-free, non-fat frozen desserts or bars; juice popsicles (freeze 100% juice in Popsicle molds); low-fat yogurt with fresh fruit

Sweet Treats

Fresh fruit, dried fruit

If you catch yourself making poor snack choices, I suggest that you come back here and look at this list. Hold yourself accountable for the snack choices you make. Make choices that will put you at an advantage here.

Step 5: Do the Right Thing at Fast Food Restaurants—Order Healthy!

Teens eat a lot of fast food. And no wonder: It's cheap, familiar, fun, and available, anytime and anywhere. What's more, it's a part of our social experience. We hang out with our friends at the mall food court or have a bite to eat down at the local Mickey D's. Or maybe you eat fast food several times a week because your mom and dad are busy. My friend Pete told me that he goes into a "fast food coma," if he doesn't get a fast food fix at least once a week. Fast food is, well, just a part of life.

So I'm not going to slam fast food and tell you to totally stay away from it. A little fast food on occasion isn't going to kill you. It's just not a good idea to eat it every single day.

Most of the major fast food restaurants now serve a lot of healthy choices. When I looked into this, I was amazed at how much healthy stuff you can actually get at these places: salads, sandwich wraps, side dishes like baked potatoes, grilled chicken sandwiches, veggie burgers, veggie pizzas, low-fat desserts, and even some reduced-fat burgers. I've included a long list for you (Supplement C) in the back of the book. Please check it out. My suggestions are based on the choices that are the lowest in calories and fat.

The Power Portion Plan: Putting It All Together

How does this plan work in real life? To help you put it all together, I've included some sample menus for you below. You can mix and match breakfasts, lunches, dinners, and snacks to get all the servings and nutrition you need every day.

And by the way, *eat breakfast!* If you do, you'll score higher on tests, have more physical and mental energy—plus, you'll have a healthier body weight (teens who skip breakfast tend to have more body fat). My dad always used to joke that breakfast was the most important meal of the day, "because if you're not home by then, you're in real trouble." But that's a whole other book. Obviously it's healthy for more nutritional reasons too!

All kidding aside, I know you think you don't have time to make and eat breakfast in the morning. But hear me out: No matter how rushed you are in the morning, you can still eat breakfast. The sample breakfasts below take less than two minutes to fix.

Also very important: Drink eight to ten glasses of pure water throughout the day. Water makes you feel full and keeps you fit and hydrated. Plus, some girls tell me they swear by it for good skin.

Power Portion Breakfasts

1. Toasted whole-grain bagel, hard-boiled egg, fresh peach, 1 cup low-fat milk. *(Portion counts: 1 power protein, 1 lean dairy, 1 fruit, 2 natural carbs—bagel counts as 2)*

2. Fast food breakfast: Apple bran muffin, scrambled egg, 1 cup orange juice, and 1 cup low-fat milk. *(Portion counts: 1 power protein, 1 lean dairy, 1 fruit, 1 natural carb)*

3. 1 smoothie, blended with 1 cup low-fat milk, 1 packet of instant breakfast mix or meal replacement powder, 1 cup frozen unsweetened strawberries. *(Portion counts: 1 power protein—instant breakfast or meal replacement powder can count as a protein—1 lean dairy, 1 fruit)*

4. 1 whole-wheat toasted English muffin with one slice of cheese, 1 cup calcium-fortified orange juice. *(Portion counts: 1 power protein, 1 fruit, 2 natural carbs—muffin counts as 2)*

5. 1 low-fat granola bar, 1 hard-boiled egg, 1 apple, 1 cup low-fat milk. *(Portion counts: 1 power protein, 1 lean dairy, 1 fruit, 1 natural carb)*

6. 1 cup whole-grain Cheerios with 1 cup low-fat milk and 1 sliced banana. *(Portion counts: 1 lean dairy, 1 fruit, 1 natural carb)*

7. 1 slice whole-wheat toast with 1 tablespoon peanut butter, 1 fresh pear, 1 cup low-fat milk. *(Portion counts: 1 lean dairy, 1 fruit, 1 natural carb, 3 healthy fats)*

Power Portion Lunches

1. Hamburger (3-ounce patty on a whole-wheat bun with lettuce and tomato), 1 cup low-fat milk, 1 apple. *(Portion counts: 1 power protein, 1 lean dairy, 1 fruit, 1 non-starchy vegetable, 2 natural carbs)*

2. Tuna salad sandwich (made with 3 ounces tuna and 1 ta-

blespoon mayo) on two slices cracked-wheat bread, 1 cup vegetable soup, 1 fresh orange, 1 cup low-fat milk. *(Portion counts: 1 power protein, 1 lean dairy, 1 fruit, 1 non-starchy vegetable, 2 natural carbs, 3 healthy fats)*

3. Fast food lunch: 1 grilled chicken salad with 2 tablespoons reduced-fat dressing, 1 serving low-fat frozen yogurt. *(Portion counts: 1 power protein, 2 non-starchy vegetables, 3 healthy fats)*

4. 1 slice veggie pizza, 1 small side salad with reduced-fat dressing, 1 cup lowfat milk. *(Portion counts: 1 lean dairy, 2 non-starchy vegetables, 1 natural carb, 3 healthy fats)*

5. 1 roast beef sandwich (2 slices lean roast beef, mustard, lettuce, and tomato on whole-grain bread); 1 cup mini-carrots with non-fat dip; 1 cup fresh grapes. *(Portion counts: 1 power protein, 1 fruit, 1 non-starchy vegetable, 2 natural carbs)*

6. 1 chicken taco (flour or corn taco, unfried), ½ cup Mexican rice, 1 cup low-fat milk. *(Portion counts: 1 power protein, 1 lean dairy, 2 natural carbs)*

7. 1 bowl meatless chili, 6 whole-wheat crackers, 1 cup tossed salad with 2 tablespoons reduced-fat dressing, 1 cup yogurt with ½ cup water-packed peaches. *(Portion counts: 1 power protein, 1 lean dairy, 1 fruit, 1 non-starchy vegetable, 1 natural carb, 3 healthy fats)*

Power Portion Dinners

1. Spaghetti (whole-grain pasta) with meatballs, 1 cup tossed salad with 2 tablespoons reduced-fat dressing, ½ cup non-fat, sugar-free ice cream. *(Portion counts: 1 power protein, 1 lean dairy, 1 non-starchy vegetable, 1 natural carb, 3 healthy fats)*

2. 3–4 ounces grilled chicken, baked potato, 1 cup cooked broccoli or other non-starchy vegetable. *(Portion counts: 1 power protein, 2 non-starchy vegetables, 1 natural carb)*

3. Fast food sub-and-soup supper: 1 six-inch turkey breast sub, 1 serving vegetable soup. *(Portion count: 1 power protein, 1 non-starchy vegetable, 2 natural carbs)*

4. 3–4 ounces steamed shrimp with cocktail sauce, ½ corn on the cob, ½ cup new potatoes or coleslaw. *(Portion counts: 1 power protein, 1 non-starchy vegetable, 2 natural carbs, 3 healthy fats)*

5. Fast food dinner: grilled chicken Caesar salad with reduced-fat dressing, ½ plain baked fast food potato, 1 carton low-fat milk. *(Portion count: 1 power protein, 1 lean dairy, 2 non-starchy vegetables, 1 natural carb)*

6. Lightly breaded fish fillet, 1 medium sweet potato, 1 cup green beans, yogurt and berries for dessert (1 cup fruit yogurt with 1 cup blueberries). *(Portion count: 1 power protein, 1 lean dairy, 1 fruit, 2 non-starchy vegetables, 1 natural carb)*

7. 3–4 ounce sirloin steak, 1 medium baked potato, 1 cup tossed salad with 2 tablespoons reduced-fat dressing, 1 cup low-fat milk. *(Portion count: 1 power protein, 1 lean dairy, 1 non-starchy vegetable, 1 natural carb, 3 healthy fats)*

Nourish and Flourish

Food is an amazing substance, really. It affects how we look and how we feel, right down to our mood, our thoughts, even how well we perform on tests. For example, I know that if I eat too much junk food, I feel sluggish, low on energy, and just kind of blah afterwards—like I'm moving and thinking in slow-mo. But when I eat healthy foods (fruits, vegetables, whole grains, and lots of water instead of soft drinks), I feel as if I could climb Mt. Everest—twice—then win a game of chess with my younger brother, Jordan.

Jay's Power Portion Plan at a Glance

- Each day, select three portions from each of the six food categories: power proteins, lean dairy foods, fit fruits, non-starchy vegetables, natural carbs, and healthy fats.
- Shoot for a total of 18 portions a day.
- Spread your portions over breakfast, lunch, dinner, and two or three snacks.
- Select a variety of Get-Full-and-Fit Foods to help keep cravings in check.
- Drink eight to ten glasses of pure water daily.
- Cut back on your intake of high-sugar foods such as soft drinks.

It's good to eat for nourishment and energy, and not restrict foods because of some new fad diet. Food shouldn't be used as a drug to deaden stress or pain. That's abusing food. Food is a tool we can use to care for our bodies.

Action Plan

Your body is your greatest physical resource. That's why it's important to give it what it needs. There are foods that work for you or against you. Focus on changing your nutrition to get better results. That's where my Power Portion Plan will help you. For a quick review of how it works, check out the box above.

- Do you have one or two foods you binge on, or eat too much of, and you know they're not really good for you?

Foods I binge on:

• Is there a healthier food you could substitute?

Substitute food(s):

_____

• Look over the Gulp-and-Gain foods listed earlier in this chapter. Try to go without one of these foods for a week. See how this makes you feel.

• When I gave up this Gulp-and-Gain food for a week, I felt:

_____

❑ Write out today what you will eat tomorrow. Stick to your plan.

❑ Promise yourself that you will use the Meal Tracker for one week.

Being overweight is no fun. Having an eating disorder is dangerous. If you can learn enough about good nutrition to make healthy choices most of the time, without obsessing over what to eat and not eat, you can make healthy changes in your diet—and in your body. You can get to a weight that's right for you, and not have to go on some serious diet. Knowing the nutrition basics here and putting them into action is a big step toward liking what you see in the mirror, feeling good, and staying healthy.

Chapter 9

Key 6: Intentional Exercise

Why You Need This Key:

To get yourself in shape, physically and mentally—and have fun doing it

I play basketball regularly. I have a lot of fun doing it because I get to spend time with my friends and compete, and I get in shape while I am doing so. Playing basketball can be as social as it is athletic. In fact, my friend Anthony and I get together and play at least a couple of times a week. Oh and by the way, I *hate* to run! It doesn't matter if I am on a treadmill, or a track, or whatever, I hate it. The whole concept of running on a track is to me, inherently contradictory. I mean think about it: If I was in such a hurry to get back, I shouldn't have left in the first place. The only time you will catch me running without a ball in my hand is if I am late to a test or if someone with a weapon is chasing me. With basketball, however, I am constantly running and seldom realize it.

If you're like me, your idea of a marathon is watching back-to-back reruns of *The Simpsons*. So before I go any further, let me clarify what this key is *not* about. It's not about training you for the Olympics, not even for next week's track meet. It's not about getting you to adopt the "no pain, no gain" mantra. And it's not about making you drag yourself to the gym six days a week. It's just not.

What this key is about is setting the controls of your life on "active autopilot," so that you love the ride and enjoy the positive rewards that flow from it.

And most of those rewards you already know, but let me re-play them for you: Being active keeps you at a healthy weight by burning up extra calories. It shapes your body and your muscles. It makes you stronger so you can ride a skateboard, nail your tennis serve, or score the winning touchdown. It improves your endurance for sports, recreation, even walking up a flight of stairs. It keeps you flexible so you can dance, play team sports, or jump on a trampoline without worrying about pulling a muscle. Basically it keeps you in shape.

But did you also know that being active:

- Weakens bad habits like overeating, smoking, or drinking alcohol.

- Increases your alertness, creativity, and concentration so you can keep your grades up and do better on tests and other school assignments.

- Gets you out of a bad mood if you've had a tough day at school, a fight with your friends or your parents, or if you just feel kinda crappy.

- Gives you a chance to meet new people and socialize with your friends or teammates.

- Builds your self-esteem by giving you a sense of achievement, pride, and confidence.

- Helps you like your body more because you're doing something good for it and with it and feeling the positive results.

I am not trying nag you to death with a bunch of facts about how exercising and being active are so great, or guilt you into trying it. Not at all. I'm just bringing this stuff up to get you thinking that exercise may not be such a bad deal after all, and that it might just be cool to be fit and healthy.

The Incredible Shrinking Guy

Grant was a guy who worked at our local movie theater. I don't know if he was eating more popcorn than he was selling or what, but I bet he had a lot of trouble fitting into those theater seats. This guy could have worked a second job as the screen. I mean he was big. Then one summer, I started seeing less of Grant at the theater—and I mean that literally. The guy was shrinking. By the middle of the next school year Grant was in terrific shape. He'd lost about a quarter of himself, at least 75 pounds. I was so amazed and curious that I had to ask him what he had done to lose so much weight. Here's what he told me:

Viewing Options: ➡ view all messages ➡ view all messages ➡ outline view

UNTITLED MESSAGE

I've been big my whole life. People would stare and some-times kids would even point when I walked by. Whenever I ate, I knew that people were watching me, thinking, "He shouldn't be having that bacon cheeseburger." Once a girl walked by my table and said, "Why don't you try a salad?" I've also been called names like "whale" and "lard-ass," right to my face. It was so humiliating. It hurt, it really did. One day I just had enough. I decided to do something about it.

My dad had a treadmill and a set of weights gathering dust in our basement, so I started using them. I'd put on my head-phones and just start walking on the treadmill. Then I'd hit the weights. At first it was hard. I could barely do five minutes of walking. But it got easier as I stuck with it. The weight started dropping off. I didn't really change what I was eating. But after a while, I didn't even want the junk food I used to crave. That's the main thing I did, exercise. It just made me feel better about myself. It made me want to eat healthy.

➡ reply to this message ➡ add to favorites ➡ view all replies

As Grant found out, exercise has this amazing ability to unplug your unhealthy, self-destructive behaviors like overeating or eating too much junk food. Plus, it incinerates calories—up to nearly 500 calories for every hour of weight training or fast-paced aerobic activity like running, dancing, or biking. I'm no math genius, but even I can figure out that if you exercised an hour a day six days a week, you'd burn up to 3,000 calories, or a little less than a pound of fat (which equates 3,500 calories) in that time. Exercising six days a week is probably a little much, but this shows that you can burn quite a few calories in an hour.

Exercise is the best weight-management trick there is. A lot of experts say if you can do just one thing to maintain a healthy weight, it should be exercise. You can get your weight under control and stop worrying so much about what you eat—and do it automatically, just by getting your butt in gear.

What's Your Excuse?

Like Grant, you do have to *get moving* off the couch or away from your computer. But here's the usual problem: You want to change your lazy lifestyle or you're thinking about exercising—someday. You have to get past wanting and thinking. Because *someday* is not a day of the week. You mean to do it, but you never quite get there. Thoughts without action are, I promise you, your worst enemy.

Your natural tendency, whether you want to admit it or not, is to make excuses. You want to exercise, but you have too much homework and not enough time, or you're too broke to join the gym. It's human nature. You didn't invent this; it's the norm. Lots of people mean to exercise but don't.

Top Ten Self-Cons for Not Exercising

I asked a bunch of teens to tell me why they don't exercise. Here's what they said:

I don't like exercising.

I lose interest in exercising.

I think exercise is boring.

I'm uncoordinated.

I'm too fat to exercise.

I don't like to sweat.

I look stupid when I exercise, so people make fun of me.

I don't have time because I've got school and homework, or I've got to go to work.

I'd rather hang out with my friends, and sit and talk.

I just don't feel like moving.

How pathetic are some of those excuses? All they do is keep you from being your best. If you're using any of these excuses, it's not a good thing. Making excuses gets in the way of having an active, healthy life. That's something we're going to change, right here and now. You're going to set up your life so that your natural tendency is to be active and enjoy it so much that it becomes part of who you are.

To get there, there are a few steps that I think you have to follow. Doing so gives you a lot of power to change the way you've been living and really get in good shape. Here is some idea of where we're headed:

Make it fun: Choose an activity or activities you enjoy, including those with a social payoff, so that an active lifestyle is easy to maintain. Remember, this isn't about becoming an athlete.

Make it something you can get good at: Find out what you can do well; then build on it.

Make it challenging: Step up your effort.

Make it stick: Set yourself up for exercise success.

Make it rewarding: Use reinforcers to keep you going.

Let's get moving. These simple steps will transform your fitness forever. But remember, you can't just want it, you have to take action and do it.

Step 1: Make It Fun

Exercise shouldn't be something you dread doing. It should be fun. But too often, you start exercising because everyone says it's good for you or to get pencil-thin thighs, or ripped biceps. That's okay, but most of the time, you'll give up when your expectations of a new-and-improved you don't materialize fast enough. And as I said, we are all that way, so don't think there is something wrong with you.

A better approach is to look for the fun in exercise. *Exercise with the intention of having fun.* Remember when you were a little kid and you climbed trees, played ball, and swam just because it was fun? Think about that: That is the kind of exercise that I am talking about. Exercising doesn't have to consist of freaking aerobics classes and power-lifting routines; it just has to be something that gets you in better shape. If you have fun while doing it, that makes it all that much better. Remember what I said about playing basketball. Don't get me wrong; there is nothing wrong with aerobics classes and power lifting, if you enjoy that (which a lot of people do). So, if you are one of those people, then do that. But if you are not, then find something else.

Somewhere along the line, it became more fun to watch TV, play video games, or instant-message with friends than go outside and ride a bike. Maybe gym class at school ruined exercise for you, shifting it from something natural you did when you were younger to something you had to do for a grade (not to mention that, annoyingly, it made you all sweaty in the middle of the school day). We have to get away from hating exercise.

The first move toward becoming more active is to identify an activity that appeals to you. Find something you like to do so much that you want to keep on keeping on doing it.

When you do what you enjoy, being active becomes so much easier. Liking an activity and getting positive payoffs from it become reinforcers for sticking with it. It is easy to do stuff that you enjoy doing.

To get you moving in the right direction, let's take a time out here to complete the following Personalized Exercise Quiz. What kind of stuff do you like to do? What sounds like fun? This quiz might help you start thinking about an activity or activities that might be right for you. Remember that you should check with a health care professional before starting any exercise program.

Personalized Exercise Quiz

There are five parts to this quiz. In the parts labeled A, B, C, D, and E, select the statements that are *true for you most of the time*. Maybe the statements in Part A are more true for you; on the other hand, perhaps the statements in Part B describe you better. Think about each statement carefully; decide which ones more accurately describe you; then circle the number of each of those statements. If a statement doesn't fit you, don't mark it. So, pick each statement that accurately describes you in Part A and circle it (them); then do the same for Part B, Part C, Part D, and Part E.

Part A
1. I like stuff that brings out my competitive side.
2. I enjoy participating in team sports.
3. I play to win.
4. If given a choice, I would rather attend a sporting event than go to a party or a movie.

Part B
1. I don't mind trying the newest thing in sports.
2. I enjoy being active, mostly for the adrenaline rush it brings.
3. I like to push myself to the edge and don't mind taking a few risks.
4. I'm not afraid to try something new.

Part C

1. If given an opportunity to compete, I would prefer an individual sport to a team sport.
2. If I must exercise, I like to get into my own zone and avoid outside distractions.
3. I'm physically self-conscious and uncomfortable participating in team sports.
4. I am not coordinated enough to perform certain sports.

Part D

1. I go out of my way to be with other people.
2. I would rather work out with another person than by myself.
3. I find group activities more fun than doing things alone.
4. I'd probably exercise more if I had a few friends who would join in with me.

Part E

1. I would like to do something that is low-impact and gentle on my body.
2. I do not like to sweat.
3. Exercise should be more meditative than anything else.
4. Competition is for professional athletes.

What's Your Score?

Look over the five parts of this quiz and zero in on the statements you circled. Wherever you have the majority of statements marked, that clues you into activities you'd probably like. So, which part—A, B, C, D, or E—has the most marks?

Scoring for Part A

If most of the statements you circled are in Part A, you're competitive and play to win. Team sports or competitive games are your passion. Put that intensity to use and try some of the following:

- Any active team sport, such as football, soccer, basketball, volleyball, baseball, or softball

- Racquetball or handball

- Golf

- Martial arts

- Competitive endurance sports such as running or competing in marathons or triathlons

Scoring for Part B

If most of the statements you circled are in Part B, you're a thrill-seeker who likes to take it to the edge and push boundaries. You love to get your adrenaline pumping by trying hot sports, such as:

- Inner-tube sledding

- Ski biking

- BMX biking

- Mountain biking

- Roller hockey

- Rollerblading or in-line skating

- Skateboarding

- Surfing

- Snowboarding

Scoring for Part C

If most of the statements you circled are in Part C, team sports are not really your thing. You prefer activities that don't require too much special skill. You may also benefit from an organized routine, with specific exercises and measurable goals to attain. Activities that best suit you include:

- Weight training

- Exercise machines (treadmill, elliptical trainer, stationary bike, etc.)

- Walking and fast walking

- Jogging

- Running

- Swimming

- Biking

Scoring for Part D

If most of the statements you circled are in Part D, you really love to hang with other people. Group activities are your best bet. Gather your friends and sign up for an exercise class or train for a race. That way, you can be with your friends and get fit all at the same time. Some other great options for you might include:

- Any type of group exercise class (boot camp or spinning, for example)

- Dancing

- Weight training with a friend or exercise partner

- Group endurance activities (running or biking clubs, for example)

- Water aerobics

- Team sports that you can all be involved in (basketball, volleyball, soccer, etc.)

Scoring for Part E

If most of the statements you circled are in Part E, you're the private type who treasures meditative time, where the only person you have to bond with is you. If you're self-conscious about your body right now, you should consider exercising in the privacy of your own home or bedroom, using exercise videos or a home weight-training set. You may also prefer low-impact activities that emphasize flexibility and are conducted in a quiet atmosphere designed to bring about inner stillness. Some options to consider:

- Yoga

- Pilates

- Tai chi

- Stretching

- Hiking

- Home exercising

This quiz has been designed to help you pick activities you enjoy. Maybe though, you discovered that there are a bunch of activities that appeal to you, from sports to exercise classes to weight training. This is a good thing, because it means you can vary your activities to provide a change of pace and prevent boredom from setting in.

If you have marks in several areas, then try out the suggested exercises from each area, see what you enjoy the most, and then go from there.

Fitness and Friendship

So far in this step, we've looked at how to choose exercise you enjoy. Another ingredient in making exercise fun is including time to be with your friends. It's the social payoff you get from exercise that can be powerfully motivating. You didn't have to score high in Part D to get this fringe benefit of exercise, either. Here's what I'm talking about:

- **The companionship you feel when going to an exercise class with your girlfriends.**

- **The teamwork and support you get when shooting hoops with your buddies.**

- **The connection you make working out with your girlfriend or boyfriend.**

- **The social skills you build by being on a team, in a race, or in an exercise class with friends.**

Try It, You Might Like It

There are so many ways to make exercise fun—and you don't even have to do it with other people. For example, you could dance really hard for 20 minutes to your favorite music, right in your own room, by yourself. That would be a really great workout, and it would be fun!

I hope this step opened your mind to the possibility that there are activities out there that will work for you. It is always easier and safer to stay on that couch and never try anything new, because

> The easiest way to get in shape is missed by most people because it is dressed in sweatpants and looks too much like work.
>
> —Jay McGraw

then you can never screw up or be disappointed. But it's definitely not as rewarding. And what's the worst that could happen? If you try basketball and absolutely hate it, you don't have to do it again. But what if you love it? If you don't try, you may never know. So if you're feeling nervous about leaving your comfort zone, the next step will help you get over it.

Step 2: Make It Something You Can Get Good At

Any activity you're considering must be something you have the physical ability and coordination to do, or believe you can master. Rollerblading might sound like a lot of fun—until you fall smack on your tailbone for the hundredth time because you have no balance and just can't get the hang of it. Or going down a mountain on your bike may be a cool idea, but not for someone who's generally cautious by nature.

I knew a girl in high school who just wasn't cut out for sports. She could barely stand on Rollerblades, couldn't catch a ball to save her life, and never even learned how to ride a bike. Games like tennis and softball just weren't for her. But you know what? One day she starting lifting weights and doing yoga (which don't require a lot of athletic ability). You wouldn't even believe the results. My totally uncoordinated friend now has the body of an athlete—

she's lean and toned and is probably in better shape than most people I know.

Forcing yourself to do something that's too hard for you or a little on the scary side does nothing but bring on needless anxiety and frustration. You've got to feel the "I-can-do-this" spirit in whatever activities you do. The greater your *can-do,* the stronger your *will-do.*

Let me tell you about me: The things I can do well, and the things I can't. I can't sing (I've been asked to *not* sing at karaoke). I can't dance either. I have tried and I just end up hurting myself and anyone close to me. It isn't pretty. So things like cardio-funk classes (yes, guys do this stuff) are out of the question for me.

But I excel at certain sports, and basketball is one of them. Being good at basketball started with my passion for the game and the realization at age 10 that I had pretty good aim.

But just because you're better at some things than others doesn't mean you're automatically a pro. Getting good at something takes practice. From the time I was in fifth grade I worked really hard at being a good basketball player. I attended summer basketball camps, played in youth leagues, and worked for endless hours on my fundamentals in the driveway with my dad. I learned how to move to make the perfect lay-up, but only by missing so many times. So when I made the high school varsity team, I fulfilled a dream of mine because I had worked hard to get good at something I really loved. On the other hand, I'm a disaster at soccer and baseball, and predictably I hate playing both of those sports. I enjoy basketball because I am pretty good at it, but I wasn't very good the first time I picked up an orange ball. It took work. But I am really, really competitive, and so I practiced a lot so that I could win.

Bottom line: Your motivation multiplies when you know you can succeed at something. It gives you the incentive to put in the time and effort to get there. That's why there's so much truth in the old saying, "Practice makes perfect." Don't expect to be great the first time you try it, but do pick something that you enjoy practicing and that you feel you can work on and improve.

Step 3: Make It Challenging

Once you've got some positive momentum going—you're exercising at something you like and something you're getting good at—you've got to gradually ramp up to make your exercise more challenging. Maybe you can only play half-court games at first, but eventually you have to start playing full-court games. Or instead of running one mile, increase it to a mile and a quarter. If it is not challenging, it is not beneficial. In other words: Do more to get more out of it.

Here's where your goal-setting skills can make a big difference. If you've been exercising at a certain level and you're getting really good at it, it's time to set the bar a little higher and strive to leap over it. In other words, set new, more challenging goals for yourself. For example:

- If you've been going to a spinning class with your girlfriends twice a week, now make it three or four times a week, or set the resistance on your bike a little higher.

- If you've started a walking program, get yourself a pedometer. (It's an inexpensive gizmo that counts the number of steps you take.) Clamp it on to your belt or waistband during your exercise walks to help you increase your daily number of steps. Or just walk farther, four laps instead of two, or a mile and a half instead of just one mile.

- If you've mastered running for one mile without a break, try for a 10 percent increase for the next week, or try to shave a few seconds off your time.

- If you're lifting weights a few times week, maybe you're ready to increase the number of reps or sets for each exercise, or up the weight.

While we're on the subject, I want to get it on record here and now that I'm a huge proponent of weight training. According to a lot of experts who deal with teen obesity and eating disorders, lifting weights is one of the best ways to improve your body image, boost your self-esteem, manage your weight, and get fit. I weight-train, not because I want to audition for the next *Terminator* movie or bust out of my shirt like the Hulk, but because it makes me feel good—and good about myself.

There are a lot of different ways to train with weights, and both guys and girls may benefit from it. To help you get started, I've included some important guidelines for you in the box "Getting Started on a Weight-Training Routine."

Whether it's weight training or something else, whatever intensity you're putting into it, demand more of yourself the next time you do it.

I really enjoy weight training, but I am not just talking about pumping iron. You or your parents might not feel that it is safe for you to lift heavy weights, and that could very well be true. In fact, many doctors say that weight training, if done improperly, can be harmful to young kids whose bodies have not yet developed enough and thus are not prepared to lift weights.

Something else that I do both for variety and for safety, and something that I really recommend and encourage you to try is working out with elastic resistance bands. Those same doctors that frown upon weight lifting highly recommend using these bands as a safe alternative to weight training.

These bands are great because they are safe, they are effective, and best of all they are cheap enough and small enough that you can use them at home. Look up these bands on the Internet because they are a really great and safe way to work out.

Whether you are working out with old-fashioned iron or the resistance bands, take a look at the table below for some great tips on starting a weight-training and muscle-building routine.

Getting Started on a Weight-Training Routine

- Begin by working out two to three sessions a week, from 20 minutes to an hour.
- Warm up your muscles first by pedaling 10 minutes on a stationary bike or walking, either on a treadmill or just around the block.
- Learn the basic weight-training exercises, like the leg press or squat, bench press, biceps curls, triceps pressdown, lat pulldown, shoulder press, and crunches for your abs. Ask an experienced weight trainer to show you the ropes.
- Practice correct form—no fast, jerky movements or lifting ridiculously heavy weights. The best results come from proper form.
- Perform three sets of 8 to 12 repetitions (or "reps") of each exercise. Start with a light weight, and increase the poundage slightly with the second and third sets.
- Perform one to two exercises for each body part.
- Write everything down. Write down your workout routine so that you don't forget which exercises to do. (It really is easy to skip something if you don't write it down.)
- Keep a progress chart of when you worked out, what body parts you worked out, how much weight you used, how many

reps you did, and which exercises you completed while working out. (See the workout diary in Supplement D.)

- Lift and lower the weight slowly and deliberately; fast jerky movements can hurt your joints.
- Allow at least one day off between workouts of the same muscle groups to let your muscles rest and recover.
- Don't rely just on weight training to improve your fitness. You still need to condition your heart and lungs by doing some aerobic exercise, such as fast walking or jogging, at least three times a week for 30 to 45 minutes. If you're short on time, try to squeeze in a cardio workout after your weight-training session.

Step 4: Make It Rewarding

A great way to set yourself up for success is to give yourself rewards. Rewards are positive reinforcers. So promise yourself that if you meet your exercise goals for the week, something good will follow. Reward yourself with a true treat—something you don't often do for yourself. Your rewards should be things that make you feel physically attractive, emotionally uplifted, or spiritually inspired, or be a present to yourself that is just plain fun. And that is the key: Find a way to make this fun. Rewards can be a great way to do just that. But your reward should not be a double-fudge sundae, a stuffed-crust pizza with everything on it, or food-related in any way. That would only defeat the whole purpose of getting fit and making healthier choices. So, no food-based rewards.

There are any number of rewards you can give yourself: a new DVD or workout gear, a pedicure, or an inspiring book—whatever has meaning for you. If you can't afford something right away, set aside a little money each time you exercise to save for something you really want.

If you're having trouble getting out of "lazy blob" mode, let me tell you about another type of reward system. One of the ways you can get yourself moving, even if you don't feel like it, is to tell yourself something like: "If I want to go to the movies, then I have to exercise first." Why would you exercise? So you can go to the movies and have some fun.

You've tied your desire to do something desirable (going to the movies) to something less desirable—exercising.

Your parents use this behavioral psychology on you all the time. How many times has your dad said something like, "You can watch the MTV Movie Awards tonight, but only if you do your homework first." If you don't do your homework, then no TV. You may whine and moan, but you'll do your homework if you want to watch the show badly enough. He's motivated you to study by sweetening the pot. You can pull the same trick on yourself.

After exercise has become a positive habit, you won't need to reward yourself. Why? Because exercising and the payoffs you get from it become your reward.

Another thing you can do is make a deal with yourself that you will just put on your running shoes, sweats, and jacket. That's it. After that, you can stop if you want. Ninety-nine out of a hundred times, once you've gone that far, you just work out because you're already halfway there.

Or tell yourself you just have to go outside and walk for five minutes, and if you don't feel like it anymore, you can stop. Five minutes into it you're already enjoying it, and the hard part—getting started—is over. Try these things. A lot of the time the hardest part is getting started, and this will help you get the ball rolling.

Step 5: Make It Stick

You've already begun setting your life up to make it more active: You've got tremendous momentum going for you. Everything you're doing is giving you exercise success, so that you don't have to rely on willpower to drive you. But you might have to develop some additional strategies so that negative moments or thoughts don't suck you back into a lazy lifestyle. To help you, try these solutions on for size.

Planning

When I was in high school, my mom would always make me clean my closet. So I'd hang my clothes on hangers and organize my shoes, and other junk on racks, instead of having it all piled up and cluttering every inch of the closet. Afterwards, I was always amazed by how much more space I had and how much quicker I could find stuff when my closet was organized. Our lives are like that: We have a lot going on, but we have more time than we think if we would just get organized.

Look at ways to organize and rearrange the amount of time you spend on homework, chores, part-time work, and family activities. Maybe finding more time means breaking your date with the TV remote, limiting the time you spend at your computer, or spending a little less time at the mall.

Another thing that helps me is to not multitask so much. I used to always watch TV and do my homework at the same time. It took forever, and I did poorly at both. Finally, when I decided to just do my homework and then watch TV later, I did better on my homework and I got to watch more TV.

Once you have made some extra time, then make an appointment with yourself to exercise. Carve out time in your schedule, several times a week, every week, to do it, and mark it on a calendar if you need to. Keep your exercise appointments just like you do with your other appointments with the doctor or with your hairdresser. Don't let anything interfere, absolutely nothing. You're more likely to stick to it when you have a regular schedule.

There's another way you can plan: by making your world "exercise-friendly." Have cues (reminders) to exercise around you—your exercise clothes in plain view, a treadmill or stationary bike in your room, or a route home that takes you by your gym—to make it easy to fall into exercise with as little trouble as possible.

Progress Report

As I said earlier, keep a workout diary that tallies up your achievements—the miles you've walked or jogged, the weights you've lifted, the exercise classes you've attended, or the number of times per week you've played sports. A personal record-keeping program (where you tell the truth!) can give you really important feedback on your progress, and keep you "on task" and working toward the goals you've set. In the back of the book, I've included a sample workout diary for you (Supplement D) that will help you keep track of your progress.

Partner Up

Make arrangements to work out with a motivated friend. You're less likely to duck out on an exercise session if your friend is counting on you to be there. Or get involved on a team. Same deal: You wouldn't want to let your teammates down by not showing up. It is easy to just skip a day here and there on your own, but if skipping a workout means standing up your friend, then you are much less likely to skip.

Having a friend will help you get a leg up. Ultimately though, no one engineers your success but you.

Prioritize

Prioritize being active into your life as something important and fun. When you do that, it means that you commit to following through. It means you make the time and devote the time because being active has taken on a special significance for you.

Don't be a slacker. If you start telling yourself: "I have to exercise before I e-mail my friends," then the difference in your rate of progress will be amazing.

Being active is just another way of putting yourself at the top of your priority list. And there's nothing wrong with that. If you don't take care of yourself, then it won't get done. The better you take care of yourself, the better your life goes—mentally, emotionally, socially, spiritually, and, of course, physically.

Moving . . . and Moving On

You have now been introduced to some incredible new steps to becoming more active. This exercise thing isn't necessarily about getting a perfect body (although it does help you get in healthy shape and stay that way). It's more about feeling good in the body you've got. It's about making your body work better so you can feel more self-confident, release the stress of all the craziness in your life, improve your body image—and most of all, have some fun.

Action Plan

Being active has so many more positive payoffs than just getting in shape. When you do something you enjoy, you'll find that exercise can actually be fun. Getting in shape while having fun—now that's a pretty cool combination.

- What's your biggest excuse for not exercising?

My excuse: _____

My plan for getting past this excuse: _____

- Of the activities I talked about in this chapter, which ones do you like best and would like to try? Pick three.

Three activities that sound fun to me:

_____

_____

_____

- Decide that you will start your exercise program today, with at least one of these activities. Make a promise that you will stick with it for at least two weeks, exercising at least three times a week for about an hour each time. See how you feel after two weeks.

How exercise makes me feel:

_____

_____

_____

- Rewards help keep you going. What are three non-food rewards you can give yourself for sticking with your exercise program?

Ways to reward myself:

_____

_____

_____

Your body is designed to be active. Keep it in good working order. When you do, you won't have to worry so much about what you eat or what you look like. Exercise frees you from these things and makes you feel great about yourself.

Chapter 10

Key 7: Your Circle of Support

Why You Need This Key:

To surround yourself with people who will boost you up so you can reach even your highest goals.

don't remember this story because it happened to me when I was a runt, but my parents have told it to me so many times, I feel as if I remember it. It was 1979, the year I was born. I was barely three weeks old, when the doctors diagnosed that I was suffering from something that could kill me. The valve to my stomach had squeezed shut. I needed immediate surgery, or else I would starve to death.

My dad didn't admit it until years later, but he was horrified, not by the illness, but by the idea of putting me, a newborn, to sleep for surgery. As he describes it, "At that age, it's real easy to go to sleep and not wake up."

He insisted on being in the operating room with me. Not only that, he insisted on keeping an eye on the drugs that the doctors used in order to put me to sleep for the operation. Mom told me, "He was going to be in there with you—no matter what."

Obviously, I woke up and lived to tell about it. But the reason I bring up this story now is to show you that everyone needs champions, people who will stay in their corner, be there for them, go to bat for them, support them, and stand up for them. My mom and dad have always been there for me when I needed them, and I've never forgotten it. When you have champion-level support in your life, it's so much easier to achieve your goals and become the person you are meant to be. That's what this key is all about: building a circle of support—people who can be of the greatest help to you because they believe in you and care enough to help you win.

Your Circle of Support

You probably already have champion-level support in your life, maybe more than you realize. This quick exercise will give you a chance to identify those champions in your life and see all the great ways they support you. On the other hand: You also have to figure out who's not on your side, and how those people may sabotage you, or work against you, intentionally or unintentionally. Once you know who those people are, you can learn to respond to their sabotage and deal with their interference. Sometimes, you can even turn saboteurs into champion-level supporters.

For starters, I want you to think about the people in your life—people you know and who know you. These can be your parents, grandparents, brothers, sisters, other relatives, friends, schoolmates, teachers, a minister, a coach, a doctor, employers, and other people who have influenced you. Now that you have these people in mind, read and answer the questions on the next page, filling in the blanks with these names.

You may want to do this exercise in your journal to keep it private. If someone's name turns up on a couple of questions, that's okay. This is not intended to give you a list of "good guys" and "bad guys." Nor is this a slam book, like some people pass around at school just to be mean. It's for your eyes only. The idea is not to cast blame, but rather to help you be aware of who's in your corner and who's not.

None of these people who turn up on your list is ultimately going to give you what you need to be successful. Only you can do that. But you will see the quality of their friendship and support in the way they react to the positive changes yet ahead of you.

As we go forward, please realize that getting help with stuff is not a sign of weakness. Everybody who is really successful has a group of supporters who help and advise them. So let's build your circle of support.

1. Who can give you good advice about nutrition, healthy eating, and exercise? _____

_____

_____

_____

2. Who will eat the way you want to eat to help you stick with your program, or offer to exercise or play sports with you when you ask? _____

_____

_____

_____

3. Who will compliment you when you're working hard to improve yourself? _____

_____

_____

_____

4. Who will drop everything if you need help?

_____

_____

_____

5. Who will stick up for you if other people tease you?

_____

_____

_____

6. Who will make fun of you when you try to get in better shape? _____

_____

_____

_____

7. Who will make negative comments?

_____

_____

_____

8. Who will get jealous or mean when you start to be successful or look better? _____

_____

_____

_____

9. Who will say things like "You'll never do it" or "You can't do it"? _____

_____

_____

_____

10. Who will pressure you into breaking your healthy routine and doing unhealthy or otherwise self-destructive stuff? _____

_____

_____

_____

Scoring

Look over the names of the people you listed in questions 1 through 5. These people make up the circle of support you already have in your life. Don't get hung up on how many people there are. A circle of one or two true champion-level friends or family members is worth more than twenty or thirty acquaintances. The quality of support is much more important than the quantity.

Look over the list of people you named in questions 6 through 10. Your answers here represent the saboteurs around you, and the areas in which they hurt your progress—with peer pressure, name calling, or other negative influences. Again, don't worry about numbers here, because you're going to learn some great tools for dealing with these people. Just realize that you may not be able to count on their support because, from the outside, the positive changes you're making look scary and feel threatening to them. They may be jealous of what you're trying to do because they can't do it, and that makes them feel bad about themselves. They may feel inferior, so they tear you down to falsely build themselves up. It all adds up to them trying to hold you back, to their way of thinking and doing, because they don't like it when you change or try to change. They want you to do what they do and conform.

The Power of Peer Pressure in Your Life

A lot of the people you listed above might be your peers—the people you hang out with because you have things in common, you like the same stuff, or you are in the same grade, for example. Within a group like this, we are usually very vulnerable to peer pressure because we feel the need to fit in and be accepted. Peer pressure can make a really smart person just like you stop thinking for yourself and get totally sucked up in what's going on around you. That's why a lot of teens go through vicious hazing, join gangs, or become part of destructive groups like bulimia cliques, where all the girls are into throwing up or taking laxatives to control their weight.

In peer groups, what we do, how we act, the decisions we make are based on the brainless creed: "Everybody else is doing it." Normal, natural, well-meaning human beings start doing the dumbest and most self-destructive acts I've ever seen all because "everybody else is doing it."

I hate to tell you this, because I know that you already know this, but the fact that "everybody else is doing it" is a lame reason for doing anything. It completely overrides common sense and good judgment. What are we thinking, anyway? If we are caving in to peer pressure to do drugs, pig out, sleep around, blow off school, or defy our parents just because everyone we hang out with is doing it, we have stopped thinking. Peer pressure can also be a good thing in the form of study groups or support groups for various problems, but even in these situations we need to think for ourselves.

I'm not trying to lecture you or tell you what friends you should or shouldn't have. All I am saying is that being part of a group can be either a good experience, if those friends help and support the decisions you make, or a bad experience, if those people just expect you to be part of the herd, which is never going to provide any real success. You have to be responsible for the consequences that come from choosing to follow the crowd. You and your friends may do stupid stuff together; we all do. But when it comes time to pay the price for stupidity, you pay for it alone.

My opinion is that if you want to be independent, if you want to be your own person, then do it. Don't just say it. I mean truly, no kidding, bottom line, be who you really are. Think for yourself. Choose for yourself. This key will help you.

Action Steps

Understanding the power of peer pressure and knowing that some people will try to hold you back are important steps, but they aren't enough. You need to have a plan of action to respond to these things. Because your circle of support is so critical to your success, we are also going to talk about how to pick the right team to help you do what you have to do. The person with a plan almost always comes out ahead. I am really big on having a plan, so let's create one here for you.

Step 1: Have a Peer Response Plan

Sometimes it's tough to recognize how people are sabotaging you, because after all, it's coming from people who are supposed to be your friends, people you trust. But you can be sure you're being pressured when your friends say things like:

"Everyone cool is doing it."

"You're an idiot if you don't do it."

"What's wrong? Are you scared to try it?"

"If you want to hang out with us, you'll do it."

I know this sounds dorky and clichéd, but it is true. Think of some more examples of phrases like this. If you at least acknowledge to yourself that this is peer pressure, and it's real, then you have a huge advantage. It seems weird that just knowing this can give you an advantage, but if you can anticipate it and prepare yourself by deciding ahead of time what to say to deal with the pressure, then you are much more likely to make good decisions. What works best is a simple "No, thanks. I don't drink" or "Nah, I don't eat Baskin-Robbins anymore," spoken calmly, but with honest force. It's tough for someone to argue with a simple "no." After all, what part of "no" is so hard to understand? Another trick that I always use is to give a reason like "Bathing suit season is coming up" or "I just ate; I'm not hungry" or "My parents would kill me."

Then, follow up your "no" by suggesting an alternative activity, such as "Why don't we go to a movie instead?" or "How about a game of basketball?"

Be kind when you can, but firm when you have to. You are the only person responsible for what you eat or drink, or what you do to get in shape, and if the people in your life don't get this, then that's their problem, not yours. You have to be very careful not to let other people in your life keep you from reaching your goals. You can be sensitive to their fears and help them to a degree, but you need to let them own and be responsible for their own feelings. Do not do things that are bad for you just to please someone else. This is about you; it is not about them.

Keep in mind that some of the people you hang out with are just not going to change their ways; but you can certainly change your reaction to them. Think about it: You can rarely change other people. But what you can change is yourself and how you react. Your girlfriend might not stop asking you to go get ice cream, but you can certainly start saying no. The first person that you need to demand change from is you. When you stand up for yourself and for your right to have what you want, you may find that people in your life will stop bringing you down because you've shown them that they can't. No one has the power to make you give up on your goals unless you let them.

Step 2: Make Peers Your Partners

Rob is a fun, popular guy at his high school. He was a running back on the football team, an honor roll student, and an outgoing person with a great sense of humor, and he had friends in every grade.

One summer, Rob gained a bunch of weight—and it wasn't muscle—mainly from sitting at a computer all day, handling website and e-mail traffic at his dad's real estate office. But with football season coming, he knew he had to get back in shape. It wasn't going to be easy, since a lot of his close football buddies were big eaters and fast food fanatics. But true to form, Rob put a funny spin on his weight-loss efforts. He had a T-shirt printed up for himself, which he wore whenever he went out to eat with his friends. The T-shirt said *Please don't feed the animal.*

When it became clear to his football buddies that Rob was serious about getting in shape, but that he was approaching it in a funny, nonthreatening way, they responded by being really supportive. Not only did they "not feed the animal," they got into the act and went for turkey sandwiches and Diet Coke instead of nasty, greasy, double-bacon cheeseburgers and shakes at fast food restaurants. (By the way, the football team was a lean, powerful fighting machine that year, and they made it to the state championship.)

Just like Rob, you've got to stay determined, but at the same time, try some humor to help break the ice with people you think might not cheer you on. You may be able to win over your high-pressure friends if you add an element of fun and creativity to your support building. Rob was a great example of what I'm talking about.

Step 3: Rise Above the Sabotage

There is an ugly side to people that I wish didn't exist, but it does. So let's just dig it up and try to tolerate the stench. Sometimes people are mean. They can call you names, act nasty, and try to leave you out—and they'll do it to your face and even in front of other people. It's five hundred times worse if you're dealing with a weight problem. People at school may call you fat, ugly, stupid, or lazy. Some of them won't hang out with you; they may totally ignore you and act as if you don't even exist, or not sit with you at lunch or in class. You probably already know this—maybe because you've been there. And it stinks.

This kind of treatment—I call it verbal violence—is an extreme form of severe sabotage, and it can have severe consequences, right down to your health and how you take care of yourself. It can make you hate your body. It can lead to dangerous dieting, even to eating disorders. It can negatively shape your self-image and make you feel miserable to the core—*but only if you let it get to you*. Read that again: Only if you let it get to you.

So how do you *not* let this verbal violence get to you?

A really, really important thing to grasp is this law of life: *You teach people how to treat you*. You do that by how you conduct yourself and the reactions you have to how others conduct themselves. If someone at school is taking potshots at you, or excluding you from a group or activity because you're overweight—guess what—you may be rewarding that behavior, however, unintentionally. Because, if you weren't, that person wouldn't continue to do it.

Maybe you acted scared around that person. Maybe you came across as vulnerable by staring at the ground and walking with a slump in your shoulders, or by some other defeated behavior. Or maybe you sent the message that you like the negative attention because it's better than no attention at all. Bottom line: People are reacting to you based on how you conduct and present yourself to the world.

(There is one exception to this law, and that's if you're dealing with someone who is really off base mentally and needs therapy or worse. If someone is rude and inconsiderate, that's one thing. If they are physically, mentally, or emotionally abusing you, that's another. You did not teach them how to do that. If someone is doing that to you, get confidential help. Talk to a counselor, pastor, teacher, or other adult.)

We can't control other people, but we can control how we react to them. Whatever your behavior, the good news is that you can choose to change it. You can choose to act differently and present yourself differently and when you do, you will get a different response. Here are some strategies you can use to teach people how to treat you:

Ignore the Comments

Or as calmly and clearly as possible, tell the person to stop it. Then simply walk away. These tactics rob tormentors of their "fun."

Deflect Comments With Humor If You Can

When you can genuinely laugh at yourself, then you won't give the other person the response he or she is looking for. If somebody says, "You walk like a duck," respond with something like, "Oh, thanks, I've worked really hard on that walk." Make your humor kind and gracious; never show contempt, or make it sting.

Convey Confidence Through Your Body Language

A great line of defense is the self-confidence offense. Walk with your head held high and your shoulders back. Look people directly in the eye in all your encounters. When you treat yourself with dignity and respect, you send a loud and clear message that you are now in a position of strength and power. If you don't treat yourself with dignity and respect, then no one else will. You may be overweight but that doesn't make you a bad person. Remember that, and a lot of the attacks will stop.

Adjust Your Attitude

The fact that people pick on you proves nothing about you. It only proves something about them. You've got to stop worrying about what everyone else thinks of you and start caring about what you think of yourself.

Put Things in Perspective

When people pick on you, it's usually because they feel inferior to you. Their self-esteem is in the toilet, so the only way they know to make themselves feel better is to put others down. People smart enough to look different or think different are easy targets. But isn't it stupid for a bully to think that trashing someone else builds him up?

I had a friend in high school who was a straight-A student, wrote for the school paper, and played on the varsity soccer team. Some tough-guy degenerates at school were making fun of him for being smart and athletic and for being a Goody Two-Shoes because he would never smoke and drink with them. My friend's dad gave him some advice—it was actually a mental picture—that really helped him. The advice went like this: "The next time they give you a hard time, imagine where they'll be in twenty years, and then imagine where you'll be. They'll be the guys parking your car, son. They aren't cool; they're losers and they know it. They're picking on you because they resent you. Just look at them and smile, because in twenty years, they'll be begging you for a tip."

Don't Give Your Power Away

If someone decides not to include you or like you, you've got to decide that that's okay with you. You must decide how you feel about you and how you define yourself. Don't give that power away to anyone else, and I mean nobody—not friends, girlfriend, boyfriend, family—nobody. If you happen to like someone, then put in some effort and energy, but don't beat yourself up if the person doesn't like you, and don't kick up your heels too much if the person does.

Stick Up for Other Friends Who Are Being Teased

This reaction teaches people that you're someone who does not tolerate name calling or any kind of verbal violence. It shows that you have integrity and would never stoop as low as putting down other people.

Even though you may not currently see how to, or believe that you can, change the way others treat you, make the decision right now that you will not give up and accept any treatment that you don't want. You do have control. You do teach people how to treat you.

Step 4: Create Healthier Friendship Experiences

If all else fails when it comes to peer pressure, there is a default position. What I have to say here will be hard to accept, but I'm going to say it anyway: During the time you are working on your weight or recovering from an eating disorder, you may have to find some new friends, or at least hang out less with the ones who pressure you to do dumb things. Changing your social life may be the best solution to resisting negative peer pressure.

You need people who believe in you and people you can count on. If your friends can't do that, then you need to surround yourself with people who will. It is your right to choose those people who will be around you while you work on yourself; you have this right and you need to claim it—no apologies necessary.

Champion-level friendship involves investing in the success and well-being of each other, no matter what the circumstances. A relationship based on anything else is dangerously limited and doesn't help you or your friend.

Step 5: Make Parents Your Partners

Let's change the channel here, and start talking about your parents. Your family can be the ultimate support system, but only if you put as much into the relationship as you hope to take out. What this involves is communication, communication, and yes, you guessed it—more communication. Your parents aren't mind readers, even if it seems as if they should be. You have a responsibility to talk to them, calmly, without fighting, about what you want and expect, and what you're looking for so that you can tap into their support to help you achieve your goals.

This isn't always easy. A lot of times there will be resistance, at first. Any time you try to change in a way that requires more from another person or takes away from something that person used to enjoy, there will be resistance. For example, if you decide to eat healthy, others in your family might feel guilty (since they should probably slim down too) or they might not understand your goals. Your mom might insist that you eat what the family eats, or your grandmother might be offended because you used to devour her homemade peanut butter cookies.

In this step, I am going to show you how to make your parents your partners so that they'll begin to support you and your goals. You'll be glad to know that this is a tantrum-free process. No shouting. No screaming. No door slamming. None of that here, so you can relax and take off your boxing gloves. The following are a few steps that could make this entire process much easier with your parents.

Clue Your Parents In on Your Health and Fitness Decisions

If you've decided to start an exercise program, or if you want to eat healthy, tell them. If you're afraid they'll talk you out of it or blow you off, say, "I want to get your input on this, but I also want to make my own decisions. I'm going to be on my own pretty soon, and I've got to start doing that. But I'd really like to know what you think."

Then really and sincerely listen to what they have to say. It's a great way to connect to your parents. The more you listen and talk to each other, the stronger the connection gets. An open ear tells them that you have an open heart. And that is important because remember we are talking about building a support circle.

The point here is to try to get them involved in your life. If they haven't been there before, this might help draw them in a little. Why would you want to do that? Because whether you admit it or not, or even know it or not, you want them there, and sooner or later you're going to need them there, cheering you on to reach your goals.

Open Negotiations With Your Parents

Your mom might make the world's greatest fried chicken, but since you want to eat healthier, you'd like it baked. Your dad wants to have three flavors of ice cream in the freezer at all times, and you would prefer sugar-free Popsicles. You may be at odds with your parents over these issues and others; how can you come to terms?

Negotiate—just as you do when you're trying to get a later curfew, or as your parents do when they are trying to get a good deal on a new car. Negotiation is all about reaching a settlement or agreement that meets the needs of both of you. The goal is to create a win-win resolution so that both sides are satisfied that they've been heard and treated fairly.

To negotiate a win-win situation with your parents, you have to come up with an agreement that you can both be excited about, and committed to. A well-negotiated agreement leaves both parties feeling that, all in all, they came out with some of what they wanted without having to give away a lot. Every deal that you negotiate with your parents needs to be a win-win deal. In other words your goal should be to make a deal that is good for both of you and meets the needs that each of you have. So, if you are going to get what you want, you have to give them what they want.

Let's take a look at a discussion where negotiation is needed:

Kim (Teen): Dad, I want to join a gym so I can get in better shape.

Mark (Dad): How much does the membership cost?

Kim: $750 a year.

Mark: That's a lot of money. How do I know you'll stick with it? I hate to spend that kind of money if you're not going to follow through.

Okay, let's take an intermission here. Is this conflict negotiable? Sure, if both sides approach it with an understanding of each other's needs. Which reminds me, before you can even meet someone's needs, you have to first figure out what those needs are. Let's look at the needs in the last conversation:

- **Dad's need is to spend money wisely.**

- **Teen's need is to get in shape by joining a gym.**

If you were this teen, you'd have to realize that Dad needs to know he's not throwing away his money. You'd have to reason with each other. Maybe Kim and her dad agree that she'll pay him back part of the membership fee if she quits. Maybe that's your negotiation. Or maybe she agrees to buy a monthly membership at first—and stick with it, so that she can prove to her dad that she is serious and deserving of a full-year membership.

There are dozens of ways to resolve conflict. The key is make your needs clear to your parents, understand what their needs are, and meet their needs by structuring your agreement so that *both* sides have obligations that can be met. When you are willing to meet the needs of another person, your needs will be met too. There are very few situations that cannot be resolved by this type of negotiation.

Inspire Confidence and Trust Through Predictability and Require These From Others

Show your parents that you're serious, not through words but by your actions. People learn by the results that you choose to give them, and in that respect, you are in control of every relationship you have.

Remember the law of life I mentioned above—that we teach people how to treat us. Well, that idea is very true and very applicable here. Have you ever heard the law of physics that says "For every action there is a reaction"? That is true with our friends and parents too.

My dad always, and I mean always, told me (and read this in a parental tone), "Jay, when you choose the behavior, you choose the consequences." Man I got sick of hearing that! I hate to say this, particularly in print, but the fact is he was right. Now, this can be good news or it can be bad news because if we act like immature idiots, then our parents will treat us like immature idiots. But the good news is that if we act like responsible, mature, young adults, then we will be treated like responsible, mature, young adults. So, we get to choose how people treat us, and that is good news.

Now, since we are talking about forming a circle of support, we should recognize that this idea works both ways. What I mean is, suppose someone has taught you through her actions that she is not going to support and help you. Then you need to not hang around with her. At least for now. I know that it sounds harsh to say this, but you should do it. Plus, chances are, as soon as you teach your friends that you won't accept anything other than their total support, then they will probably give it to you. If not, then they weren't your friends in the first place.

Let's return to our previous story to illustrate what I'm talking about. If Kim's commitment to exercise at the gym fizzles after a couple of months, and she's spending her afternoons with her computer instead of with the weights, then Kim has taught her dad that she can't stick with anything for very long. What do you think will happen the next time Kim wants her dad to cough up money for something? Not good. Kim has taught her dad that she is not committed to what she promises and that she can't be trusted. If you don't like the way that your parents or your friends are treating you, then you need to teach them to treat you differently. The choice is yours.

Step 6: Create Accountability

Accountability is something we talked about under goal setting, but it is worth repeating here, since it is so important to building your circle of support. Accountability is actually nothing more than a fancy "buddy system." You team up with someone you trust in your circle of family and friends, and make a pact that you will support each other, by working out together, and encouraging other healthy habits.

Review the questionnaire you just filled out earlier in this chapter. Now go to one of your supporters—someone you trust—and ask that person to be an accountability buddy who will call you on it and make it impossible for you not to achieve your goals. Make it a point to check in with each other during the week to see how things are going, talk through problems, and bounce ideas off each other. Try to replace your struggles with strategies.

Always remember that it is your job to achieve your goals; it is your accountability bud's job to help and support you. Your buddy can help you and make the process easier, but ultimately, only you—and you alone—are responsible for your choices and your success.

You should be proud of yourself for coming this far and going through all of these steps with me. It can be a challenging and scary process to stand up to people who try to bring you down and even more difficult to deal with their sabotage. This is a process that many people will never even try. It is great that you are taking a stand for yourself, resisting negative peer pressure and rising above it. You have begun to build a way of life that supports what you want on every side. Now go out there and have some fun!

Action Plan

A huge part of success is having people in your life you can count on—and they can count on you, because it works both ways. These people are your circle of support.

- If you want support, you have to give it too. When we help other people, it takes our mind off your own problems. Think of one of your friends who might really need your support right now—and do what you can to provide that support.

Someone who needs my help:_____
Ways I can support this person: _____

- Are you being influenced by negative peer pressure right now?

Person or people who are pressuring me: _____
My peer response plan for this situation: _____
_____
_____
_____

- How you act determines how your parents and peers treat you. Treat yourself well so that others will be motivated to do the same. What are five things you can do this week to start treating yourself better?

1. _____
2. _____
3. _____
4. _____
5. _____

- Identify something you need to negotiate with your parents in order for you to get in better shape and achieve your fitness goals.

Your need: _____
Your parents' need: _____
What are some ways both needs can be met?

_____

_____

_____

So what can a circle of support do for you? Lots. The most important thing is that it moves you closer to your goals and helps you achieve them. Having this circle and being accountable to each person in it means you will get in better shape, you'll have more fun with your friends because there will be less peer pressure, and you may even get along better with your parents in the process.

Chapter 11

If You Have an Eating Disorder: Applying the Seven Keys

nap! It sounded like an explosion. You could hear it throughout the entire gym. Kerrie screamed out in pain: "Ahh, my leg! Somebody do something!" It was painful even to watch, one of those sights that make you sick to your stomach. Kerrie, a very accomplished high school gymnast, a girl who had colleges lining up to give her scholarships, was landing a string of hand springs and flips, the final sequence of her floor routine that would clinch the regional championship for her team. Then it happened: Her leg broke so badly that I could watch the agony on the video her mother had shot on their Handycam.

Kerrie was not doing anything that every gymnast doesn't do. Nothing should have gone wrong, but it did. It went really wrong! She fractured her femur, one of the strongest and biggest bones in the body. Thankfully, there was a paramedic team on hand, as is always the case at high school gymnastic meets, that could rush her straight to the emergency room.

It was there at the hospital, talking to the doctor, a woman perplexed at the break, a woman who was telling the family how uncommon it is to break a femur, that Kerrie's parents, Jim and Marci, learned of the horrible fact that their daughter was suffering from an advanced case of bulimia. The doctor was the first person to ever ask Kerrie about her eating disorder, the first person to bring up the subject so taboo that Kerrie avoided it at all costs.

"Kerrie, do you have an eating disorder?" The doctor asked point-blank. Kerrie looked up, focusing on something other than the excruciating pain for the first time since the break. This sobering question allowed her to focus just long enough to know that this was the time to fess up. "Wh . . . why do you ask?" she stuttered.

The doctor knew exactly what was going on and explained to

the family that when someone develops a severe eating disorder, her body becomes emptied of the necessary vitamins and nutrients required to keep bones strong and healthy. She explained that usually when a young, thin girl came into the ER with a bad break, it was probably due to an eating disorder.

I recently talked to Kerrie about the horrible experience that required numerous operations and a very uncomfortable cast to get her walking again.

Viewing Options: ➡view all messages ➡view all messages ➡outline view

UNTITLED MESSAGE

I knew that what I was doing was bad for me. I knew that it was going to catch up with me someday, either because my teeth were decaying, or my esophagus was being damaged. I even thought about breaking a bone some way, but no matter how much I wanted to stop, no matter what side effects I learned of, I couldn't make myself stop. I cannot stand having a mass of food in my stomach. This means throwing up my food because I want to feel empty and cleansed inside, with a flat stomach on the outside.

Throwing up gives me this real sense of control over my body. It feels good afterwards. It is a feeling that I really can't fully describe, but I guess I felt a sense of mastery, no one could control that aspect of me except me, and I liked that. It was a feeling that I wasn't willing to give up.

➡reply to this message ➡add to favorites ➡view all replies

As Kerrie continued to speak to me, what began to unravel was the story of how her lifestyle completely revolved around her disorder:

Viewing Options: ➡view all messages ➡view all messages ➡outline view

UNTITLED MESSAGE

I weigh myself as soon as I get up in the morning, without any clothing. Socks and underwear can give a false reading. I make sure my feet are placed in a certain position on the scales so that I get the most precise reading. What the scales tell me is very important to my emotional state on any given day. If my weight is up, I feel very depressed, and it is hard to focus on school and other things. If it is down, then I am happy, and I congratulate myself. I've been successful, and I eat even less than I ate the day before.

When I get to school, I make it a point to walk as fast as I can to get from class to class, because I know that being on the move will burn more calories. I don't eat lunch. Instead, I use the time to walk outdoors on the paths that encircle my school.

There are times when I get depressed and so I binge, and eat tons of cookies and sweets. A friend told me that what goes into the stomach first, goes out last.* So I am careful to eat a food like a red apple, or something with a skin, at the beginning of a binge. Something bright that I can see on the way out. That way, I know when my stomach has been fully emptied of everything I've eaten.

At night before I go to bed, I weigh myself again. I want to make sure that I didn't gain any weight during the day. And if I did, I must be even more careful the next day.

➡reply to this message ➡add to favorites ➡view all replies

* This is a myth. What goes into the stomach first doesn't necessarily come out last, since the stomach mixes everything around.

Starve Wars in America

Kerrie is one of millions of Americans suffering from an eating disorder, and like these millions, everything in her world seems to center around the disorder. The two most common of these disorders—and the two we will focus on here—are anorexia and bulimia. Anorexia is a desire to be so thin that the sufferers of this disorder literally starve themselves. If you have this disorder, weight is most likely something you feel you can control in a world where it seems as if everything else is controlled by others. Extreme dieting, purging (throwing up or taking laxatives), and excessive exercise are some of the main methods used to control weight. But no matter how thin you get, you still think you're too fat.

Bulimia involves eating tons of food (bingeing), followed by purging, usually through vomiting or taking laxatives. It very often begins with a diet and a desire to control your weight, but eventually becomes a way to medicate moods. With bulimia, food and purging become ways to soothe stress, release pent-up anger, or fill some other emotional hole.

Eating disorders now rank as the third most common chronic illness among female teens. At least 50,000 individuals will die each year as a direct result of an eating disorder. Tragically, anorexia is now the number-one cause of death among young women. Death comes calling usually in the form of organ failure.

I talk and write a lot about teens in crisis, and eating disorders clearly represent a huge crisis among youth today. I am not an eating disorders expert or a doctor, but I have had close friends who have suffered from eating disorders. I have seen the pain, and I have seen the devastation it brings to young lives.

For me to write this chapter and give you all the thoughtful knowledge and guidance you deserve to have, I brought in the "cavalry." That cavalry is my father, "Dr. Phil," and his friend and mentor, G. Frank Lawlis, Ph.D., one of the country's most respected psychologists. Both have worked extensively with people who have had eating disorders, and with their families, to help keep these illnesses from wrecking lives.

What you will have on these pages is the gift of their wisdom, knowledge, and guidance on how to treat these very distressing and deadly disorders. In addition to working with my dad and Dr. Lawlis on this chapter, I surveyed thousands of teens, asking them about eating disorders and weight. My job is to take what I have learned from all these valuable resources and translate it into information that will be healing for you.

If you have an eating disorder, you might think that it is too big a problem to overcome. Yes, it is a big problem, but it is not a hopeless situation. There is light up ahead.

First Things First: Let's Get Real About You

Before we go any further, let me ask you something: Do you actually have an eating disorder?

A lot of us diet, overeat, binge, or try to sweat off a hot fudge sundae in the gym, on occasion. But that doesn't mean we've got an eating disorder. It's only when these things start to dominate our lives and push all healthy, rational activities out of our lives, that they become an eating disorder.

What I'd like you to do is take a few moments to answer the following questionnaire, which was put together by Dr. Lawlis just for this book. It will help you acknowledge whether you have a problem, so that if you do, you can begin to change it. Answer all twenty questions as truthfully as you can by checking one response for each.

		Yes	Sometimes	No
1.	Are you terrified of losing control of your weight?	—	—	—
2.	Have you gone on eating binges and not been able to stop eating?	—	—	—
3.	Regardless of how much you weigh, do you *always* see yourself as fat or getting fatter?	—	—	—
4.	Do you feel that any kind of food you eat will turn into fat on your body?	—	—	—
5.	Do you feel that you have no other tools for controlling your weight other than not eating or vomiting your food?	—	—	—
6.	Do you feel that the only way you can be attractive is to be thin?	—	—	—
7.	Whenever you look at yourself in the mirror, do you see a fat person?	—	—	—
8.	Do you feel extremely guilty or panicky after you eat?	—	—	—
9.	Are you preoccupied with thoughts of food most of the day?	—	—	—
10.	Do you frequently go on diets, restricting your food intake to lose weight?	—	—	—
11.	Do you fight to maintain self-control around food?	—	—	—
12.	Do you use laxative, diuretics, or diet pills for weight control?	—	—	—

	Yes	Sometimes	No
13. Have you ever considered suicide?	—	—	—
14. When people tell you that you are attractive, do you believe them?	—	—	—
15. Do you become resentful and angry when you deny yourself food?	—	—	—
16. Do you go on binges when you get depressed or angry?	—	—	—
17. Is your self-worth completely attached to how slender you are or how much you weigh?	—	—	—
18. Have you ever vomited to control your weight?	—	—	—
19. Was there a special moment or event in your life when you were told that you were unattractive and you have believed it since?	—	—	—
20. Do you normally use exercise or activity to burn off calories you've just eaten?	—	—	—

Scoring

For every "Yes," score a 2; for every "Sometimes," score a 1. Add up all twenty responses to arrive at a sum ranging from 0 to 40.

What Your Score May Mean

0–3   Mostly likely, you do not have an eating disorder. However, pay extra attention to items you marked "Yes." These might be red flags for something you need to stop doing or thinking.

4–12   You may have some eating disorder thoughts and attitudes. Maybe you're overly afraid of getting fat, or you feel guilty about eating. You might have experimented with purging, restrictive diets, or excessive exercise. These thoughts and activities can be self-destructive if allowed to continue.

13–20 You may be down the path to a serious eating disorder, where you are obsessed on controlling your weight in unhealthy ways.

21–30 You have symptoms of an eating disorder, and you should seek professional help.

31–40 Your eating disorder has most likely become an illness that requires medical and psychological attention, especially if these behaviors and thoughts have persisted for six months or more. You need to be under the care of a psychological and medical team.

The Seven Keys to Freedom From Eating Disorders

If you are barreling toward an eating disorder, or suffering from one now, you are in danger. Some of you may even be dying. My hope for you is that you are reading this chapter because you know you are in trouble, you're ready to stop denying it, and you want help. You only have this one life to live. Why not make it the best it can be? This chapter—and the seven keys—can help rescue you.

As we revisit the keys, I do not intend to delve into the deep, dark reasons why you have developed an eating disorder. You may be wondering how in the world you ever got started down this path in the first place. There are many very complex reasons behind eating disorders: growing up in a critical family, childhood sexual or physical abuse, depression and hostility, low self-esteem, pressure to be slim, negative feelings about your body, even genetics. Sometimes, though, the "whys" just can't be answered.

I'm not saying that you shouldn't give some time or thought to these things; you should. But you've got to get busy fixing this problem: If all you did was focus on why you have an eating disorder, not taking any other action, you could starve yourself to death or die of a heart attack. A lot of these circumstances you can't change. But you can sure change what you do with them *now.* The solutions lie within you—the choices you make, the actions you take. Using the seven keys, taking them to a deeper level, will help you find the solutions you need. We are not going to just review the seven keys in this chapter, but rather, we are going to talk about how to directly apply these keys to overcoming an eating disorder.

Key 1: Right Thinking

You have already done a lot of work on changing your self-defeating, or "bully," thinking and replacing it with reality-based right thinking. However, some of your thoughts may still seem really hard to bust loose from your brain. You've got to keep working at Key 1, using the Truth Test in that chapter to challenge your assumptions. Try keeping a thought diary in which you record your thoughts, challenging their truthfulness and helpfulness in writing, and where you create uplifting, productive alternatives. Doing this will help reinforce better thinking habits.

I want to be extra clear on certain points that I feel are big deals when it comes to right thinking and eating disorders.

Labels

Labels are names you call yourself. Many of these labels either came from within you when you saw yourself messing up in life, or they have come from other people. But whatever their source, we tend to internalize these labels, believe these labels, and live by these labels. They can become the definition of you if you let them.

Go on alert to the label of "anorexic" or "bulimic" in your life. These are labels that can slow down your progress and wash away your sense of self. You are not defined by these disorders. They are problems that can be conquered; they are not your identity.* Make the choice to get rid of labels that limit you in any way.

The Debate Within

Do you ever feel as if there are competing, debating voices going on inside your head? Imagine the debate team residing in your brain, only there are two of you, your "Bully Self" and your "Healthy Self." The Bully Self eggs you on to do negative things, while the Healthy Self—the part of you that knows better—tries to resist. This inner debate has a huge influence on you. If one side wins, the other side loses.

Some days the Bully Self is stronger and just seems to take over, and some days the Healthy Self has the upper hand. No, you're not going crazy. According to therapists who treat these disorders, many people who struggle with food and weight-related issues have this debate within. Here's what it sounds like:

---

* You are Sara or Mark or Sue or Andy or Tami and you are dealing with an eating disorder. You are not "a bulimic" or "an anorexic."

Healthy Self: I do not want to binge today. Leave me alone. I don't need you bugging me.

Bully Self: Yes, you do.

Healthy Self: Why?

Bully Self: Because you really want to eat that package of Oreos. It will make you feel better.

Healthy Self: No! I want to make good nutritional choices and exercise with my friends.

One way to deal with this debate is to bring it out into the open and be aware of what's going on inside you. Write down in your journal the debate that goes on inside between your Bully Self and your Healthy Self. Writing this down is important, it really drives home the need for change.

But it is also important to reinforce the power of your Healthy Self and muzzle your Bully Self forever. What are you most proud of?

In the list below, check off any items that describe you. Then add to the list yourself. Write down any characteristic, quality, or achievement that gives you pride in being who you are—that's your Healthy Self.

_____ I can love deeply.

_____ I am a good friend to my friends.

_____ I am fun to be around.

_____ I am smart.

_____ I have volunteered for important causes that I believe in.

———— I am creative.
———— I have a special talent or gift.

_____

_____

_____

Keep going. You haven't even scratched the surface yet. Acknowledging all the good, special characteristics you have will help you get in touch with the inner beauty that is you—and board up your Bully Self for good.

Body Image Distortions

Some of the loudest and most damaging inner dialogues going on inside you involve your body image, that mental picture you have of your body. Teens with eating disorders often have very negative body images. Sometimes how you feel about your body can infect how you see yourself as a person.

Learning to accept and love your body is something else that takes time. But there are some simple steps, practiced over and over, that can help you.

Pay Less Attention to the Media

Remember that these images of "beautiful people" are very distorted and electronically manipulated to look thinner or more buff. They are not real. You are real.

Be Kind to Your Body

On a more regular basis, take more time to pamper yourself. This can involve massaging lotions into your skin, having makeovers, getting manicures or pedicures, or taking long bubble baths. Don't avoid touching your body, either; this may only keep your self-hatred of it alive. You must learn to love your body, and this is one way to do that.

Think About Your "Heroes"

We all have heroes—the people we respect and admire the most. It could be a teacher, a relative, a friend, a parent or grandparent, someone in the news, or someone who lives on in history. Right now, list five people you consider heroes, people you personally admire and respect. There is only one rule here: The people on your list cannot be superthin.

Beside their names, list the qualities that impress you the most about these people. These can be their intelligence, integrity, self-confidence, personality, style, achievements, and so forth.

My Heroes   ## Why I Admire Them

1. _____   _____

                                 _____

2. _____   _____

                                 _____

3. _____   _____

                                 _____

4. _____   _____

                                 _____

5. _____   _____

                                 _____

Now, look at the qualities you listed for your heroes. Ask yourself:

Do I have any of these qualities?

What can I do to develop them?

Do I think being thin or in shape is the highest priority for the people who are worthy of hero status in my life?

What do I think is truly important to these people?

To help change your body image, you need to realize that people who have success, fulfillment, and joy in their lives do not measure their self-worth by their appearance.

Eat Right, Think Right

There is one more thing to recognize with this key. Poor nutrition and self-starvation will disturb your thinking. You'll have poor concentration. You'll have trouble making decisions. You'll feel more stressed-out than normal. You'll be emotionally out of whack because of a lack of nutrients to your brain. What is so important to do is to start making the right nutritional choices as soon as you can, with the help of Key 5. It can be life-changing to work on your self-talk. But that is of no use if your brain cannot process normally. Once you start nourishing yourself physically, it will become easier to talk to yourself the right way. All the keys work together. They give you the power to make your life better.

Key 2: Healing Feelings

Eating disorders are not just problems with food or weight. They are also a cry for help or relief—an attempt to use food or weight to deal with emotional problems. One of the best ways you can heal your feelings is to go through the step-by-step process that we talked about in Key 2, from understanding how perceptions affect your emotional life to the importance of getting emotional closure on emotional pain.

Remember that our emotions—like fear or anxiety—are based only upon our perceptions of what is happening to us. The interpretations we make of the events of our lives, and the reactions that we have to them, are all that matters. In other words, no matter what happens in your life, how you interpret those events is up to you. It's our interpretation of things—how we think about them—that disturbs us, not the things themselves.

A lot of teens with eating disorders interpret their situation with an attitude of fear. They have an intense fear of being fat. They panic around food or about having to eat in the company of other people. They are afraid of losing control. Or they fear change. Sure, it's normal to be anxious and afraid, but you can't let yourself be dominated by fear. Feelings of fear keep you paralyzed, pessimistic, shut down, and insecure. You've got to stop giving your power away to fear.

How to Conquer Your Fears

If you panic at the thought of food, eating out with people, gaining weight, or giving up control, it is because you've got some thoughts flashing through your brain at lightning speed. These are thoughts that you've talked yourself into believing, such as "I'll get fat if I eat," "I'll eat too much if I eat out with people," "I'll gain weight if I have to stop purging." Such thoughts are so well rehearsed and stamped on your mind that they are practically automatic. All you have to do is register "food" or "eating," and you immediately think "bad deal" and become unglued.

What you need to do is to put your mind into slow motion like a video or film. Then listen to what you're telling yourself, and challenge those beliefs. Close your eyes and recall times when you got stressed-out by food, eating with other people, or whatever situation brings on your fear. Listen to what goes through your mind. Write it down in your journal. Next, challenge your beliefs. Just as you learned in the chapter on Key 1, apply the Truth Test.

In nearly everyone who has an eating disorder, there is the fear that giving up the eating disorder will cause them to spin out of control. Has this fear infected your own thinking? If so, challenge your fear of losing control. Is it really control to not eat? Is it really control that your life revolves around your eating disorder? Is it really control to avoid going to a restaurant with your friends because you are afraid of being around food? The truth is, you're not in control; your eating disorder is. Challenging your fears like this helps stop the behaviors that flow from them.

Sometimes, overcoming fears means exposing yourself to what you're most afraid of. For example, if you're scared of situations related to eating (like eating at a restaurant) because those situations make you anxious, you need to come up with a plan to get over this. You might eat out at a restaurant with someone in your circle of support, someone who is helping you overcome your eating disorder. Next, you might go to a restaurant with a couple of supportive friends. From there, you might "graduate" to going to a party where there is food. You must continue to go through this process until you've done it so often that you're no longer afraid of what you've been avoiding.

Learn to challenge the fears that have their hooks in you. When you do, you'll lift yourself up to a place where you can see all kinds of possibilities for yourself.

Key 3: A No-Fail Environment

With this key, you took some super-important steps to set your world up for success. You started getting rid of cues to binge or purge, like controlling your access to binge foods, laxatives, and diet pills. You went on the alert for people who could be obstacles to your getting well. You've done all this so that when your enthusiasm conks out, your environment will support you.

But maybe right now, you need a little something extra. After all, eating disorders can lock you into rigid, fixed patterns of living—patterns that are hard to shake loose.

Maybe you've heard the joke about the teen who for lunch every day ate a tuna fish sandwich, and every day she complained to her friends at the lunch table about how she hated tuna fish sandwiches. One of her friends got so sick of the constant complaining that she said, "If you don't like tuna fish sandwiches, why don't you tell your mother to fix something else?" To which the teen replied, "Hey, don't bring my mother into this. I make my own sandwiches!"

You may be laughing at that teen, but I'm telling you, that's you. To change your life, you've got to put a different filling in your sandwich. When you choose how you live, the more fun, the more fulfilling, and the more successful your life will be. So start now. Shake it up!

Here are a few suggestions for breaking out of your fixed patterns—just to prove that you can do it. Make a deal with yourself: Change one thing in your environment every day for the next couple of weeks. Start with some of my ideas, but add some of your own. For example:

- Rearrange your bedroom.

- Change your hairstyle.

- Change your wardrobe, trying some new combinations of clothes.

- Change the time you get up in the morning, or go to bed at night.

- Play different music.

Add some ideas of your own. In the space below, list five additional changes you can make to shake up your environment.

1. _____
2. _____
3. _____
4. _____
5. _____

The point here is to break from the old and come in with the new. When you begin to do different things, your actions pick up speed. Your life gains positive momentum. This paves the way for victory.

Key 4: Mastery Over Food and Impulse Eating

Changing the behaviors, or choices, that are a part of your eating disorder may be one of your biggest challenges because they've become habits. You're hooked on whatever payoff the behavior is serving. Starving may give you the payoff of control. Bingeing may be a way to deaden pain. Purging may be a way to release anger or stress.

You have to ask yourself whatever the payoff is, is it really what you want, or are you hiding from life? I mean, think about it: Can you throw up, starve, or take laxatives to really fix your problems and cope with life? No way! These behaviors are draining you of the critical life energy you need to go after things you truly want.

It is real important that you continue to uncover the payoffs that are driving these self-destructive behaviors. Only then will you be better equipped to make the changes you most want to make.

Break the Cycle of Destructive Behaviors

Many of those changes involve the habitual behavior patterns you've gotten into as a part of your eating disorder. If you think about those patterns, you may find that they are very rigid, repetitious, and predictable. A typical pattern, involving thoughts and actions, might look like this:

You get stressed-out.

You go on a binge.

You feel scared of getting fat.

You vomit.

You fast for the rest of the week.

Each one of these behaviors, choices, and thoughts is like a link in a necklace. Each one leads to, and links up with, another. But if one link is broken, the next one—the next behavior—usually won't happen. Take vomiting, for example. For many people with eating disorders, the urge to vomit after eating can have a pull as strong as a magnet. In eating disorders, vomiting is one of the main behaviors that keeps binge behavior going. If someone with anorexia or bulimia knows she can vomit after a meal or binge, she'll keep on vomiting. On the other hand, if opportunities to vomit are taken away, or the behavior is stopped, she'll be less likely to binge. So breaking links in the necklace is a good way to stop self-destructive patterns altogether. Here is what Hailey, age 19, told me about her experience.

Viewing Options: ➡ view all messages ➡ view all messages ➡ outline view

UNTITLED MESSAGE

I had an eating disorder for six years, from age 12 to 17. The last year of my disorder, I was purging several times a day by vomiting. By that time, I was in therapy. I remember during one session, my therapist made this one suggestion. She said, "I want you to agree to try to stop the vomiting. Binge if you have to, but don't vomit." For the longest time, I didn't try it. I was too afraid of gaining weight. But then one day, I binged big-time on nachos and ice cream sandwiches. Normally, I would have puked it all up. But I was just so sick of myself, sick of hanging over the toilet, sick of vomit burning my throat, that I decided to not throw up. I felt stuffed, bloated, and very uncomfortable from the binge. In fact, the discomfort was worse than the discomfort of vomiting. But I didn't purge. I had a few more binges that week. But again, I didn't purge. I just sat around feeling sick, bloated, and yucky, every time. Over the next couple of weeks, I had gotten so disgusted by the physical effects of bingeing that I stopped bingeing. So in less than a month, I had stopped purging and I had stopped bingeing. The whole thing was kind of a miracle. My therapist explained to me that I had disrupted the chain of binge eating and purging. I don't care how she explained it, it was still a miracle to me!

➡️reply to this message ➡️add to favorites ➡️view all replies

---

What Hailey just described about vomiting can apply to any type of self-abusive behavior that occurs in a pattern. You have to remove the opportunity. My dad once counseled a patient, "If you want to throw up, you must do it in the living room in front of everyone else." That nipped that behavior in the bud pretty quick.

The point is: You must make a heartfelt decision to stop the self-abuse. Put your mind to it—and do it. If it helps, then create a schedule such that the activity that you are trying to avoid is impossible to do. For example, if you always throw up after you eat the plan is to start eating where there is no private bathroom available. It might also be easier to create a new, incompatible behavior than it is to get rid of the old habit. For example, if you can't make yourself stop throwing up, then make a deal that you will no longer go to the bathroom alone. If you go, someone else goes with you. This new behavior is pretty much incompatible with throwing up and may be a good way to break that habit.

Knowledge Is Power

I believe that knowledge is power. The more you know about the consequences of doing something, the better your choices to either do it or avoid it. That's why it helps to have a few facts about these behaviors. Here's what my medical advisors told me:

- **Vomiting isn't even an effective way to control your weight. More than half of the calories you eat from a meal or binge are absorbed by your body. So you're not really getting rid of all the food. Vomiting, of course, damages your teeth, throat, and esophagus, plus causes a disturbance in your body's mineral balance that can lead to heart trouble.**

- **Laxatives have very little effect on calorie absorption, and diuretics have zip. What's more, abusing these rather powerful drugs can really mess up your insides and again, lead to mineral balance disturbances that can be life-threatening.**

Reality check: These things don't work as weight loss tools. They don't prevent your body from absorbing calories. Instead, they make you sick. Understanding this sometimes makes it easier to quit these behaviors.

Healthy Substitutes

Take every opportunity you can to break out of the behavior ruts you're in. As I said earlier, one of the best ways is to use the strategy of incompatible substitutes that we talked about in Key 4. Incompatible substitutes are activities, like relaxation, listening to music, calling friends, or writing a letter, things that are incompatible with bingeing or purging.

Keep a list of your incompatible substitutes with you all the time. Add to and change this list from time to time, noting which activities worked and which ones did not. But the key is that when you feel the urge to binge, purge, or starve, take out your list and start doing one or more of your alternate activities. With a strategy like this in place, you'll be less likely to cave into the urges when they hit.

Key 5: Jay's Portion Power Plan

Nutritionally, the single most important move you can make now is to set up a pattern of regular meals and snacks. What this means is that you eat three meals each day, with two to three snacks—preferably at set times during the day.

If you can make a commitment to do this, you will find that your self-destructive eating and food behaviors will start to gradually fade away. Remember that to get rid of one habitual behavior, you've got to replace it with a new behavior that is incompatible with the one you are trying to eliminate. Scheduled eating is incompatible with bingeing, starving, or other forms of food chaos. If you break this link in the chain then you have a good chance of breaking free from the entire chain.

Here is what a typical meal schedule looks like:

7:00 a.m.	Breakfast
10:00 a.m.	Snack
12 noon	Lunch
3:00 p.m.	Snack
6:00 p.m.	Dinner
9:00 p.m.	Snack

In the space below, create a meal schedule for yourself that fits your day.

_____   _____
_____   _____
_____   _____
_____   _____
_____   _____
_____   _____

Here are some additional guidelines to help you get started.

Use the Portion Power Plan to Figure Out What to Eat at Each Meal and for Snacks

This plan gives you the freedom to make healthy choices, without resorting to obsessive calorie counting. Make sure you have healthy foods on hand, and shoot for 18 portions a day.

Try Not to Skip Meals or Snacks

Skipping a scheduled meal or snack can invite bingeing or starving. If you are tempted to eat between your scheduled meals or snacks, grab your list of incompatible substitutes that you constructed in Key 4, and start doing something on the list right away.

Preplan Your Meals

Writing out what you will eat for the day helps prevent binges and sudden impulses to overeat. When you plan your eating in advance, you don't have to rely on the fickle emotion of willpower to keep you from bingeing and otherwise getting off course.

Get Back on Track After a Setback

Don't look back. Just pick up the pieces and return to your schedule of planned meals and snacks.

Gain Food Freedom

If you're like a lot of teens struggling with eating disorders and food issues, you've probably made it a point to avoid certain foods because you're afraid that they'll make you fat. Avoiding these foods, however, can make you feel deprived, which can lead to bingeing, guilt feelings over eating foods you consider "forbidden," and all kinds of counterproductive food obsessions and fears. Get over this!

What I'm about to ask you to try will seem scary at first, but it works and will help you learn to eat realistically and not be afraid of foods or give in to binges. It is especially helpful in overcoming the food fears that are a part of eating disorders.

Food Freedom Exercise

Take out your journal and write at the top: *Foods I'm Afraid to Eat.* (Of course, I'm not talking about chocolate-covered grasshoppers here—who wouldn't be afraid to eat those?) Underneath that heading, list all the foods you're afraid to eat. Some examples might be pizza, ice cream, potato chips, Twinkies, or birthday cake.

Begin to introduce one of these foods into your planned meals or snacks, a week at a time. For example, you might start by having a brownie with a glass of milk for a couple of your snacks. Concentrate on brownies for a few weeks. Then move on to another food. Keep doing this until you have built most of your feared foods in your diet and you're no longer scared to eat them. Fix normal, commonsense, and controlled servings, and eat them at the kitchen or dining room table. *Red alert:* Don't do this when you're depressed, angry, stressed, or in a situation where you feel as if you can't handle these foods.

Here's something I need to emphasize: You won't have to eat these foods forever and ever. When you're no longer afraid of them—when they no longer make you feel anxious—that's when you can cut back on them. The point, though, is not to call for an outright ban on these foods, or else you'll find yourself craving them.

Key 6: Intentional Exercise

I think we've pretty much established that exercise is generally one of the safest and easiest things you can do for your health. But sometimes, exercising can go from being intentional—something you do for fun and fitness—to excessive, crossing the line between healthy and unhealthy. In eating disorders, exercise often is used as a form of purging to burn off calories eaten from a meal or after a binge.

Exercise can also turn into a negative addiction. What can happen is this: You become so fanatically driven to lose weight that you exercise to the point where you feel you can't stop, even if you've injured yourself or you're being begged by your parents and friends to stop. Maybe you believe exercising like this will accelerate your weight loss and help you reach some unattainable body ideal. Or, pressured to succeed in sports, you think that compulsive exercise will help you win an important game. So you add additional workouts to those already scheduled with your teams, without talking to your coach first.

What about you? Is your exercise out of control? To find out, take this quick quiz, circling *Y* for yes or *N* for no to each question.

Y N   1. Are you uncomfortable resting, relaxing, or just sitting still because you think you're not burning enough calories?

Y N   2. Have you ever told yourself things like "If I don't exercise today, I'll gain weight," "If I don't run an hour, it's not worth it to even run," or "I must do 250 situps every night"?

Y N   3. Have you ever felt as if you couldn't stop exercising, that you had to keep going?

Y N   4. Do you frequently feel tired, have sore muscles, or both?

Y N   5. Do you force yourself to exercise, even if you're sick?

Y N   6. Do you get upset or down on yourself if you miss a workout?

Y N   7. Do you base the amount of exercise you do on how much you've eaten?

Y N 8. Do you worry that you'll gain weight if you miss a workout?

Y N 9. Have you ever felt that exercising is more important to you than your friends, family, school, or even your health?

If you answered yes to any of these questions, then you may have a problem. Exercise may be part of your eating disorder, and you must acknowledge this. Have the guts to say that you're be-having in a self-destructive manner, or you may not be able to get it under control. You'll continue to deny yourself into real trouble. That said, I cannot emphasize enough how important it is for you to take action. Here's some advice.

Review Your Exercise and Activity Goals

Remember that being active is supposed to be fun and keep you healthy. Don't try to change your body into some idealized shape through exercise.

Schedule Breaks, Cutting Back on Your Exercise Schedule

If your family doctor gives you a thumbs-up, you can still exer-cise, just not as much. For people with eating disorders, therapists and physicians often recommend activities such as weight train-ing, though you should always check with your doctor whether this is right for you. Weight training helps build body mass (weight) and improve body image. Other great activities are yoga and tai chi; both help relieve stress. For now, stay away from the high-impact stuff, such as jogging, running, or aerobic dance.

These burn too many calories, interfering with weight gain, and may lead to broken bones.

Focus on the Non-Weight-Related Benefits of Exercise

Think about how exercise clears your mind for studying, distracts you from the pressures of school, relieves stress, boosts your mood, and lets you enjoy your time with friends.

Key 7: Your Circle of Support

Psychologists who treat people with eating disorders agree on this point: You will recover much faster from an eating disorder if you have a strong circle of support.

In Key 7, you got in touch with those people in your life that you consider to be the closest to you—the people you trust and treasure most. Eating disorders, however, hurt relationships and isolate you from the people you love. You have probably retreated from people—and further into your eating disorder. But you are not really alone. It just seems that way because the people in your life do not know how to handle what is happening to you. They want to help you, but they feel helpless. This may come across as distance between you and them. Don't continue to hide. Don't let your eating disorder rob you of something as precious as loving, supportive relationships. You need support now more than ever. Without people to help you, you'll be emotionally undernourished. Reach out instead of withdrawing. Ask for help and support. This will help get your relationships with friends and family back on solid ground.

It is also vital that you turn to others—professionals such as therapists and doctors—for your healing to continue. A therapist is a great person to hold you accountable for what you are going to do. For example, your therapist might set up a contract with you—an agreement—where you're required to call him or her before you binge, purge, or do something else destructive. That makes you accountable on a regular basis and is a great tool for getting better. If you're afraid of what the therapist or doctor might think, or if you feel embarrassed, get over it. Reach out and do not continue to suffer in silence.

For medical reasons, your family doctor or pediatrician should also be a part of your circle of support. There are lots of medical complications associated with eating disorders, and a bunch of them can kill you. But your doctor can't help you if he or she doesn't know what's going on with you.

You might also join a support group for people like you, who have eating disorders. You may believe that you're the only person in the whole world who does the odd, sneaky stuff you do. But when you join a good support group, you'll be surprised and relieved to find out that you're not alone. You'll find people who understand you because they are like you. You'll gain strength from each other.

Make sure the support group you join has a focus toward the positive, in which its members share what is working for them, without whining, without complaints, and without excuses. If there is a spirit of negativity in the air, this can zap the joy and encouragement from the experience. When you leave a support group each time, you should feel encouraged, inspired, and uplifted. If, on the other hand, you feel down, then that's not the group for you. Drop out and find a better one.

Don't Go There: Online Saboteurs

In this key, we talked previously about saboteurs, people in your life who don't give you the support you need. By now, I hope you know how to handle yourself around them. There is, however, one more source of sabotage I have to bring up: pro-anorexia websites. These places irresponsibly dispense "tips" on how to survive on 200 calories a day, how to vomit, and how to keep from ruining your teeth, and advice called "thinspirations" ("hunger hurts but starving works"). By doing this, they fuel dangerous behavior and promote eating disorders as a lifestyle. This isn't much different than showing you a wiring diagram for how to make a bomb to kill yourself.

I promised I wouldn't preach, but if you are logging on to one of these sites, or are considering it, we have to talk. That decision is nuts, and you need to *not* go there.

It is my hope that you will begin requiring more of yourself and not just gaze into the Internet, pointing and clicking your way to disaster. You are better than that and you know it.

An eating disorder can feel like a downhill slide into despair. Overcoming it is an uphill climb. The seven keys are your tools for getting to the top. Make each of them more a daily part of your life. As you do, you will build the confidence that you can eventually succeed. Your life will get better because you made it better. And remember, you may gain a little weight and that is a good thing. I know that thought is totally foreign to you, but it is true. Being in good shape is okay; being too skinny is not okay.

Conclusion

We have come to the end of this book, but in a way, this is just the beginning—the beginning of a brand new, better way of living for you.

What we have talked about here is the real deal: that to manage your weight, you have to take charge of everything you do, think, and feel. And you have to use that control to create the "healthy you" that you deserve to be and have.

That's not to say that everything from here on out is going to be easy. It's not. You'll still have a lot of second-nature habits that you've got to unlearn—habits that can really mess up your life if you let them.

I'm not trying to kill your enthusiasm here. I am just being honest. There is still a lot of work ahead. It will take effort, action, and commitment. There may still be part of you that feels comfortable with your same old ways of being and doing. That part of you might not want things to change, and it will put up a good fight.

Have you ever walked into a movie theater after the movie starts and it was dark inside—so dark that you tripped over everyone in the row and spilled their popcorn because you couldn't see where the heck you were going? But then you found a seat and settled into it. Your eyes adjusted to the dark and you could see again.

The only thing that changed was your ability to perform in that environment. It would have been much safer and much easier to just turn around and go back to the hall, but you would have missed the movie.

The same is true here. You are currently standing outside the movie, you have your date and your ticket, and now all you have to do is walk through the door. Right now, for the first time ever, you have all of the tools necessary to succeed. It may be dark on the other side of that door and the adjustment might be a little difficult, but I promise that this movie, the story of your life, is one that you don't want to miss! It will be difficult at first, but don't give up. Every day will be easier and easier until this new way of living is just a way of life. Stick with it and in no time you will be happier and healthier than ever before.

I have told you that there will be some stumbling blocks, so let's take a look at what those might be. Preparation is the best way to defeat them.

Disappointment

Perhaps you've dreamed that once your eating problems are over, the new you will be prom king or queen, you'll get the ultimate boyfriend or girlfriend, or that your parents will stop being so irritating. Then you wake up one morning, in great shape and at peace with food and your body, and none of these things have really happened. Isn't life supposed to be perfect now?

Not necessarily. Things are not going to be exactly how you want them just because you're wearing size 6 jeans—that is not the world we live in day to day. Not everyone wants to date you because you got in shape. You won't get voted prom king or queen or president of the student council just because your butt is smaller. Your parents will still be on your case even though you run a mile without keeling over. Basically, life around you is still pretty much the same.

Disappointment hits. You may say, "What the heck? . . . Was it really worth it to do all this and have the same old life?"

Reality check: You can never, ever use things like weight loss or recovery from an eating disorder to solve problems that are not related to these things. Healthy or not, you still have the same friends, the same parents, the same everything. If you expect all your problems to magically disappear when you achieve your weight and fitness goals, you are not being real.

But if you faithfully use the seven keys, you'll continue to have much greater control over your whole life. You'll have the skills and tools to handle life's ups and downs. Just hang in there and keep using what you've learned. At this point you truly do have the ability to create whatever life you want. The fact that you are in shape won't magically change every aspect of your life, but *you* can.

Negative Mindset

If you've been overweight for a long time, maybe for as long as you can remember, or you've been dealing with an eating disorder for many years, you may have a perception of yourself as a fat teen, an anorexic, or a bulimic. This is a negative mindset of beliefs that you think are true about you.

Good news here: It's just a mindset and it does not have to be true for you. You can change it, get comfortable in your new, healthier body, and dump all that psychological baggage. You can't do this, though, until you start acting like the fit, healthy person you are. Do things like looking at your reflection in the mirror more often, enjoying the new you; facing those situations you used to fear (like wearing a bathing suit or going out to eat with friends); sticking to your exercise program to appreciate your own strength and God-given shape; and tuning into and changing your negative self-talk. When you do these things on a regular basis, you'll begin to live happily and comfortably as the new, healthy you. You have worked hard, enjoy what you have earned!

Coasting

There is a natural tendency to relax and coast after reading a book like this. Don't do that! This is not the time to sit on your butt!

What you need to be doing is to keep tabs on yourself so that unwanted behavior doesn't sneak back into your life and screw up everything you've accomplished. Your health is managed, it is not cured.

For example, if you get to your goal weight, weigh yourself at least once a week. Get back on course if your weight veers too far from where it should be. Track your meals if you see yourself sliding back into irregular eating patterns, or eating too much junk food. Keep recording your exercise progress.

I think it's a good idea for you to re-read this book too, re-taking the quizzes and going back through the steps. Continue to demand more of yourself in every area of your life. Don't coast!

Another point: It is really frustrating, but when you quit working out, you will quit being in shape. Just because you may have reached your goals doesn't mean you can stop working. It just means that it is time to go into maintenance mode.

Crisis

Unfortunately, life is not pain-free. That's just the way it is. There will be pressures, and there will be crises. It is not a matter of *if* these things hit, it is simply a matter of *when*.

During a crisis or stressful time, there is a tendency to scrap all your normal priorities. You suspend all the rules, and you tell yourself that it's okay to get right-now relief for the pain. When that happens, you shift all your momentum into reverse. You retreat back into food and unhealthy behaviors.

Your best chance to take back control is to have a plan in place for dealing with crises when they hit. The plan I'm talking about involves perfecting the coping skills you've already developed—and taking them to an even higher level for even stronger coping for what lies ahead. For example, if you've learned yoga as a way to release stress, maybe you take it to the next level and study more advanced forms of yoga and add meditation. Move yourself up the performance ladder. Or suppose you are lifting weights. You probably don't need to lift more or heavier weights, but make yourself the deal that when a crisis hits, you will still force yourself to go to the gym.

When you do this, challenging yourself to do more and have more, you strengthen your resolve and your commitment. You'll be able to overcome the tough stuff when it hits.

Reward and Punishment

Some people confuse reward and punishment, and this is a huge stumbling block. A boulder, really! It sounds impossible to confuse these two things, but it's not. For example, you might feel like rewarding yourself with a triple-fudge ice cream sundae when you make one of your weight goals. But who's kidding who, here? You're defaulting to behaviors that got you into trouble in the first place.

It is okay every once in a while to reward yourself with food if you make a good grade or achieve something that doesn't involve food. For example, the sports teams I played on went out for pizza whenever we won a game. What I'm talking about is rewarding yourself with food and eating for changing food and eating behaviors. That's not the best reward in this case.

So please don't do that. It is certainly not a reward when you have worked so hard for so long to rework your mind, body, and spirit, and then choose to make dumb choices that can wreck your progress. Consider what you're losing: All this does is erase days, weeks, and months of hard, productive work, and you're back to square one. I'm not saying that you can never again have a hot fudge sundae; just don't use sundaes as a reward for eating well.

When you reach your goals, reward yourself with nonfood gifts, like new clothes, a new CD, or a new computer game—whatever makes you happy. Take care of yourself in healthy ways, and that will do wonders for your self-confidence.

Isolation

Don't ever think that because you're doing well, you don't need to stay accountable, or you don't need help from your circle of support. You do! If you want to stay healthy, live with this motto: "A healthy lifestyle loves company." (You've heard the "misery" saying, but this one's so much more fun to live!)

Keep surrounding yourself with friends, family, and other people who have the same motto—people who boost your spirit and confidence when the going gets tough. Never dissolve the supporting team you've put together. You'll always be more successful if you keep company with like-minded people who want you to achieve your goals. Continue to seek out, and be with, people who enhance your life.

If you ever find yourself tripping over these stumbling blocks, get back on your feet by using the seven keys. When problems come up, say to yourself, "I can handle this." Actively manage your life and whatever comes with it. Then and only then will you have the freedom to do what is best for your health and well-being. This is an ongoing process, but it can be fun. In no time, being healthy will become a new way of life. Enjoy that and enjoy the benefit of your hard work.

Here is what I wish for you to be thinking, saying, and feeling as you go forward from here:

Viewing Options: ➡ view all messages ➡ view all messages ➡ outline view

UNTITLED MESSAGE

It feels good to like and accept myself again. When I get up in the morning, I'm excited for the day. I'm not ashamed of my reflection in the mirror. I like what I see, and I'm proud of who I am. I've found the power to eat according to what I need instead of being driven by self-destructive habits, impulses, or diets. I am at peace with my body, and my body responds with so much more energy and strength. I am free enough to forget about food and get on with living. Gone are my old bad habits, and I now have the time to use for productive, fun activities. Whether learning a new sport, watching my favorite TV show, reading a book, doing my homework, or writing a poem, I enjoy what I'm doing more because I am not obsessed with food, my body, or dieting. I've discovered talents I didn't know I had. I realize life won't be easy in the future any more than it is today, but I know how to deal with pressures and problems. I know how to cope with life in positive ways. I am no longer going in circles, but moving forward. I am learning to understand why I am in this world and what I am supposed to do while I am here. Every day is an adventure, and I feel happy. I am learning to live a life that means something and I finally have hope.

➡ reply to this message ➡ add to favorites ➡ view all replies

---

Make this the song in your heart.

Play it often . . . and play it loud.

You have worked hard, always remember to live with a plan and have fun!

Supplement A

Relaxation Script

Find a quiet place, like your bedroom or backyard, where you will not be bugged by anyone for at least twenty minutes. No telephone rings, no e-mail, nothing but peace and quiet.

Begin to relax by imagining that your body must fight gravity to stay in a safe and balanced position. Close your eyes and begin to escape from your pressures. Visualize a special place where you feel the calmest, such as a sandy beach or a woodland trail. Dump your worries from your mind, and begin to focus only on your breath—in and out. Seven counts in, seven counts out.

Think of this ingoing and outgoing air as cleaning out all the tension in your body and replacing it with energy. This is exactly what your breathing does: It cleans and energizes your body and mind. Let your out-breath carry things away you need to let go of—your worries, your fears, your tensions. Just allow them to be pulled out the way a water current carries away debris. You're breathing out the tension, the toxic stuff, the used-up air, and replacing it with clean, healthy, oxygen-filled air. You breathe it in and out through your lungs, but it goes everywhere in your body.

Feel your lungs expand and contract. Turn inward to your body, and visualize how the powerfully oxygenated air comes in to make your body glow from the inside. You might even feel warmer.

Continue to breathe and relax your body with each breath. If there is a special place that needs special attention, put your attention there. For example, if you have some tension in your stomach, focus on that spot and your breathing will automatically become more active there. See the tension being captured by your out-breath and carried to the outside, being replaced with strong, powerful in-breaths of strength and confidence. After just a few seconds, you might feel the stress go out, with energy and warmth coming in to replace it. Allow your breathing to do its job before moving on to other parts of your body.

Just keep breathing and allow your body to feel less stressful, and more energized. All you have to do is breathe, and your body and mind will do the rest.

As you come to the end of your breathing session, become aware of your outside world, the sounds, and how you are part of it. Realize that you are healthier and less tense. You've restored your energy. You have power and control over your inner life. You can deal with anything that confronts you, as long as you can relax and use your breathing for energy and cleansing.

Supplement B

Jay's Portion Power Plan Foods

Here's a huge list of foods you can use to get on track, nutritionally. I've placed an asterisk (*) next to the foods that are Get-Fit-and-Full Foods—those that support good eating habits.

There's another list too, made up of mainly Gulp-and-Gain Foods. Those are the foods you want to cut back on, way back, because they make you eat too fast. Plus, they make you gain weight.

Try to eat three servings a day of the foods from the six food categories we talked about in Key 5. Watch your portions too!

HEALTHY CHOICES

Power Proteins

Fish and Shellfish

* Bass, baked or broiled
* Bluefish, baked or broiled

Clams:

    Canned, drained

    * Steamed

* Cod, baked or broiled

Crab:

    Canned, drained

    * Cooked

    Imitation (from surimi)

* Flounder, baked or broiled
* Grouper, baked or broiled
* Haddock, baked or broiled
* Halibut, baked or broiled

* Lobster meat, cooked with moist heat
* Ocean perch, baked or broiled

Oysters:
    Raw
    * Cooked

* Pollock, baked or broiled

Salmon:
    * Baked, broiled, or grilled
    Canned
    Smoked

Sardines:
    Canned in mustard or other nonfat sauce

* Scallops, steamed or broiled
* Shrimp, steamed, boiled, or grilled
* Swordfish, baked, broiled, or grilled
* Trout, baked or broiled

Tuna, light or white:
    * Cooked
    Canned, water-packed

Poultry (all baked or roasted)

Chicken:
    * Chicken breast, without skin
    Canned, boneless
    Chicken, ground lean

* Cornish game hen, skin removed
* Turkey
    Turkey breast, without skin
    Turkey breast, barbecued or hickory-smoked
    Turkey, ground lean
    Turkey sausage, lean

Meats

* Beef (all cuts grilled or broiled):
    Beef ground, extra lean or lean
    Eye of the round
    Round tip
    Sirloin
    Tenderloin
    Top loin
    Top round

* Lamb (all cuts grilled or broiled):
    Chop, lean
    Rib, lean
    Shoulder, lean

* Pork (all cuts grilled or broiled):
    Chop, lean
    Roast, lean

* Veal (all cuts grilled or broiled):
    Rib, lean

* *Eggs*

Whole
Whites
Egg substitute, liquid

Lunch Meats

Bologna, light (turkey)
Ham, reduced-fat
Reduced-fat or non-fat sandwich meats

Plant Proteins

* Beans (such as kidney, garbanzo, pinto, white, black)
* Soy burgers or hot dogs
Tempeh
* Textured vegetable protein (soy burgers)
Tofu

Lean Dairy Foods

Cheese, reduced-fat or non-fat:
Brick

Cheddar
   Cheddar, shredded
Feta
Mozzarella
Parmesan, reduced-fat or low-fat
Ricotta, part-skim milk
Velveeta processed cheese spread,
     low-fat

Cottage cheese:
Low-fat 2%
Low-fat 1%

Ice milk:
Fat-free, sugar-free

Milk:
1% low-fat milk
2% low-fat milk
Buttermilk, reduced-fat
Non-fat dry milk, reconstituted
    with water
Skim milk
Soy milk

Yogurt:
Low-fat, plain, sugar-free
Non-fat, plain, sugar-free

Fit Fruits
* Apples:
   Dried
   Raw
Applesauce, unsweetened
Apricots:
   * Dried halves
   Juice-packed

* Raw
Water-packed
Bananas, raw
Blackberries:
   Frozen, unsweetened
   * Raw
Blueberries:
   Frozen, unsweetened
   * Raw
Cherries:
   Water-packed
   * Raw
* Cranberries, dried
* Figs, dried
Fruit cocktail:
   Juice-packed
   Water-packed
Grapefruit:
   Canned sections, juice-packed
   * Raw
* Grapes, raw
* Kiwi fruit, raw
* Lemon, raw
* Lime, raw
* Mangoes, raw
* Melon, raw:
   Cantaloupe
   Casaba
   Honeydew
* Nectarines, raw
Oranges:
   Canned sections, juice-packed
   * Raw
* Papaya, raw
Peaches:
   * Dried
   Frozen, unsweetened

Juice-packed

* Raw

Water-packed

Pears:

* Dried halves

Juice-packed

* Raw

Water-packed

Pineapple:

* Fresh chunks, prepared from
  raw fruit

Juice-packed, crushed, chunks,
tidbits

Juice-packed, slices

Plums:

Juice-packed

* Raw

Prunes:

* Dried

Stewed, unsweetened

* Raisins, 1 packet or 2 tablespoons

Raspberries:

Frozen, unsweetened

* Raw

Strawberries:

Frozen, unsweetened

* Raw

* Tangelo, raw

* Tangerines, raw

* Watermelon:

Diced

Piece

Fruit Juices

Acerola juice

Apple juice, unsweetened

Cranberry juice cocktail, low-calorie

Grape juice (purple or Concord),
unsweetened

Grapefruit juice, fresh or unsweetened

Orange juice, fresh or unsweetened

Pineapple juice, unsweetened

Prune juice, unsweetened

Non-Starchy Vegetables

* Alfalfa sprouts

* Artichokes, boiled

* Artichoke hearts, cooked from
  frozen

* Arugula, raw, chopped

Asparagus:

Canned spears

Cooked from fresh

Cooked from frozen

* Bamboo shoots, canned, drained
  slices

Beans:

Snap beans, yellow, canned

* Snap beans, yellow, cooked from
  fresh

* Snap beans, yellow, cooked from
  frozen

String beans, canned

* String beans, cooked from
  fresh

* String beans, cooked from
  frozen

Bean Sprouts:

Canned, drained

* Raw

Beets:

Canned

* Beets, cooked from fresh

* Beet greens, cooked

* Broccoflower, steamed
Broccoli:
* Cooked from fresh
* Cooked from frozen
* Raw
Brussels sprouts:
* Cooked from fresh
* Cooked from frozen
* Cabbage, common varieties:
Cooked, drained
Raw, shredded, or chopped
Carrots:
Canned, sliced and drained
* Cooked, from fresh
* Cooked from frozen
* Raw
Carrot juice, canned
Cauliflower:
* Cooked from fresh
* Cooled from frozen
* Raw
* Celery, raw
Collards:
* Cooked from fresh
* Cooked from frozen
* Cucumber slices
* Eggplant, cooked
* Endive, fresh, chopped
* Escarole, chopped
Kale:
* Cooked from fresh
* Cooked from frozen
* Leeks, cooked, chopped
* Lettuce, all varieties, raw
Mixed vegetables:
Cooked from canned
* Cooked from frozen

Mushrooms:
* Canned, drained
* Cooked from fresh
* Raw, sliced
Mustard greens:
* Cooked from fresh
* Cooked from frozen
Okra:
* Cooked from fresh pods
* Cooked from frozen slices
Onions:
* Pearl, cooked
* Raw, chopped
* Raw, sliced
* Spring/green
Parsley:
* Raw, chopped
* Parsnips, sliced, cooked
Peas
Green, canned, cooked
* Green, cooked from frozen
Peas and carrots:
Canned
* Cooked from frozen
Peppers, hot, all varieties:
Canned
* Raw
* Peppers, sweet, green, red,
yellow
Cooked
Raw
* Rutabaga, cooked cubes
Sauerkraut, canned or bottled
* Shallots, raw, chopped
Spinach:
Canned, drained
* Cooked from fresh

* Cooked from frozen
* Raw, chopped
* Squash, summer varieties, cooked
* Succotash, cooked from frozen

Tomatoes:
  Canned
  * Cooked from raw
  * Raw, chopped
  * Raw, whole, medium

Tomato juice, canned

Tomato products, canned
  Paste
  Puree
  Sauce

* Turnips, cubes, cooked from fresh

Turnip greens:
  * Cooked from fresh
  * Cooked from frozen, chopped

Vegetable juice cocktail, canned

Vegetables, mixed
  Canned, drained
  * Frozen, cooked, drained

* Water chestnuts, canned, slices or
    whole

* Watercress, fresh, chopped

Zucchini
  * Raw
  * Cooked from fresh

Natural Carbs

Breads and Bread Products

Bagels:
  Oat bran
  Whole wheat

Crackers, whole wheat and low-fat
    varieties

Melba toast

Breads:
  Cracked wheat
  High-fiber (Branola)
  Mixed grain
  Oatmeal
  Pita pocket, whole wheat
  Pumpernickel
  Raisin, enriched
  Rye, light or dark
  Whole wheat

English muffin, whole wheat

Muffins:
  Bran, small
  Whole wheat, small

Rolls, whole wheat

Tortillas, corn or flour

Cooked Cereals

Corn grits (hominy), enriched:
  Regular and quick, prepared
  Instant

Cream of wheat:
  Regular, quick, or instant

Farina cereal, cooked

Malt-O-Meal

Oat bran, cooked

Oatmeal

Breakfast Cereals

* All Bran
* All Bran with extra fiber
* Bran Buds

Bran Chex

Corn Bran

Corn Chex

Fortified Oat Flakes

40% Bran Flakes

Fruit & Fibre

Fruitful Bran
Granola, low-fat
Grape-Nuts
Mueslix
100% Bran
Product 19
Raisin Bran
Rice Chex
Rice, puffed
Shredded Wheat
Special K
Total
Wheat, puffed
Wheat Chex

Grains
* Amaranth
* Barley, pearl, cooked
* Bulgur wheat
* Couscous
* Millet
* Quinoa

Pasta:
Spinach
Whole wheat

Rice:
* Brown
* Wild rice

Wheat bran, raw

Wheat germ:
Toasted
Raw

Starchy Vegetables
Beans:
　Black beans
　Black-eyed peas
　Chickpeas (garbanzos)
　Great Northern beans
　Kidney beans
　Lentils
　Lima beans
　Navy beans
　Pinto beans
　Soybeans
　Split green peas
Corn
Potatoes, baked or boiled
Pumpkin
Squash, winter varieties, cooked
Sweet potatoes, baked

Healthy Fats
Oils:
　Canola oil
　Flaxseed oil
　Margarine, trans-free
　Olive oil
　Peanut oil
　Safflower oil
　Sesame oil
　Sunflower seed oil
　Vegetable oils
Salad dressings:
　Blue cheese, reduced-fat or
　　non-fat
　Blue cheese, regular
　Caesar's, reduced-fat or non-fat
　Caesar's, regular
　French, reduced-fat or non-fat
　French, regular
　Italian, reduced-fat or non-fat
　Italian, regular
　Ranch, reduced fat or nonfat

Ranch, regular
Russian, reduced-fat or non-fat
Russian, regular
1000 Island, reduced-fat or non-fat
1000 Island, regular
Vinegar and oil, reduced-fat
Vinegar and oil, regular
Mayonnaise, regular or reduced-fat
Salad dressing, mayonnaise type,
        regular or reduced-fat
Nuts and Seeds:
    * Almonds, in shell
    * Brazil nuts, in shell
    * Peanut butter, reduced-fat
    * Peanuts, in shell
    * Pecans, in shell
    * Pistachios, in shell
    * Sunflower seeds, in shell
    * Walnuts, in shell

OTHER HEALTHY CHOICES

Beverages
Club soda
Diet sodas
Fruit beverages, sugar-free
Lemonade, sugar-free
Water, bottled

Meal Replacements
Beverages (230 calories or below
        when mixed with fat-free milk)
Bars (210 calories or below)

*Soups
Beef broth or bouillon
Chicken broth or bouillon
Chicken noodle

Chicken rice
Minestrone
Onion
Tomato
Tomato vegetable
Vegetable beef
Vegetarian vegetable

GULP-AND-GAIN FOODS TO LIMIT OR AVOID

Beverages
Alcoholic:
    Beer
    Hard liquors
    Liqueurs
    Wine
Carbonated:
    All sweetened soft drinks
Fruit drinks and punches, sweetened

Breads and Baked Goods
Biscuits
Bread sticks
Brownies
Cakes, all varieties:
    Coffee cake
    Fruitcake
Cookies, all varieties
Croissants
Danish pastry
Desserts:
    Apple crisp
    Fruit cobblers
Donuts
English muffins, plain
Pancakes
Pies, all varieties

Rolls and buns, made with white flour

Taco and tortillas, fried

Toaster pastries

Waffles

White bread

Dairy

Cheese, full-fat:

    Blue

    Brick

    Brie

    Camembert

    Cheddar

    Gorgonzola

    Gouda

    Monterey Jack

    Mozzarella

    Muenster

    Parmesan

    Provolone

    Ricotta, whole-milk

    Romano

Cottage cheese, full-fat varieties

Cream, sweet:

    Half and half

    Heavy whipping cream

    Light, coffee or table

    Light whipping cream

    Whipped cream

Cream, sour

Cream products, imitation diary:

    Coffee whitener

    Dessert topping

Dips

Milk:

    Chocolate milk

    Eggnog

Evaporated, whole

Malted milk

Milkshakes

Sweetened condensed

Whole milk

Milk desserts:

    Custard, based

    Frozen dessert bars

    Ice cream, full-fat

    Ice cream, soft-serve

    Puddings

    Yogurt, full-fat, sweetened

    Yogurt, frozen

Eggs

Eggs fried in margarine or butter

Fast Foods

Bacon cheeseburgers

Burritos, all varieties

Cheeseburgers

Croissant sandwiches

Double cheeseburgers or

    hamburgers

Fish fillet sandwiches

Fish sandwiches

French fries

Fried chicken pieces

Fried chicken sandwiches

Ham and cheese sandwiches

Hot dogs

Onion rings

Pizza

Sausage or bacon sandwiches on

    biscuits or muffins

Turkey club

Fats and Oils
Butter
Margarine
Vegetable shortening

Fish and Shellfish
Fried fish and shellfish
Fried fish products, such as fish
    sticks

Fruit Juice
Apple juice, sweetened
Cranberry juice cocktail,
    sweetened
Grape juice (purple or Concord),
    sweetened
Grapefruit juice, sweetened
Orange juice, sweetened
Pineapple juice, sweetened
Prune juice, sweetened

Fruits
Applesauce, sweetened
Apricots, canned in syrup
Blackberries, sweetened
Blueberries, sweetened
Fruit cocktail, canned in syrup
Peaches, canned in syrup
Pears, canned in syrup
Pineapple, canned in syrup
Plums, canned in syrup
Prunes, in syrup
Raspberries, sweetened

Grain Products
White pastas and noodles
White rice

Gravies
Gravy:
    Canned, any variety
    From mix, any variety

Lunch Meats
Bologna
Bratwurst
Brown-and-serve sausage links
Corned beef
Ham lunch meat
Hot dogs
Kielbasa
Knockwurst
Olive loaf
Pepperoni
Polish sausage
Pork sausage
Smoked link sausage
Vienna sausage

Meats
Beef, high-fat cuts:
    Choice chuck blade
    Ground beef
    Prime rib
Pork:
    Bacon
    Canadian-style bacon
    Sausage
Variety meats (liver, brains, tongue,
    heart), panfried
Veal:
    Cutlets, breaded and fried

Mixed Dishes
Microwavable dinners and entrees,
    all varieties

Poultry

Chicken patty, breaded and fried

Fried chicken

Turkey and gravy, frozen package

Turkey patty, breaded and fried

Snack Foods

Bagel chips

Cheese puffs

Corn chips

Crackers

Popcorn in vegetable oil

Potato chips

Pretzels

Soups

Any creamy-style soup

Sweeteners and Sweets

Apple butter

Butterscotch topping

Caramel topping

Candy, all varieties

Fruit Roll-Ups

Gelatin desserts, with sugar

Honey

Jams and jellies

Marshmallows

Marshmallow creme topping

Popsicles

Sugars, all varieties

Syrups, all varieties

Vegetables

Corn, cream-style

Potatoes:

    Au gratin potatoes

    French fries

    Hash browns

    Mashed potatoes

    Potato puffs

    Scalloped potatoes

Spinach soufflé

Sweet potatoes:

    Candied

    Canned

Vegetables packaged or canned

    in sauces

Supplement C

Fast Food Choices

Check out the lists below. They're your guide to a lot of fast foods that are mostly on the healthy side. Use these lists to make better choices when you go out to eat.

Arby's
Junior Roast Beef
Salads, no dressing:
  Caesar Salad
  Caesar Side Salad
  Grilled Chicken Caesar
    Salad

Burger King
Whopper Jr Sandwich,
  no mayo
Hamburger
BK Broiler Chicken Sandwich,
  no mayo

Chick-Fil-A
Chicken Filet
Chicken Sandwich
Chargrilled Chicken Sandwich
Chargrilled Deluxe Chicken
  Sandwich
Chicken Salad on whole wheat
Chargrilled Chicken Cool Wrap
Spicy Chicken Cool Wrap
Hearty Breast of Chicken Soup
Salads:
  Chargrilled Chicken Garden
    Salad
  Southwest Chargrilled
    Chicken Salad
  Side Salad
  Carrot and Raisin Salad

Dairy Queen

Grilled Chicken Sandwich,
   no cheese
DG Homestyle Hamburger
Grilled Chicken Salad,
   fat-free Italian dressing
DQ Fudge Bar, sugar-free
DQ Vanilla Orange, sugar-free
Lemon DQ Freeze, ½ cup

Hardee's

Grilled Chicken Sandwich
Regular Roast Beef Sandwich

Jack-in-the-Box

Hamburger
Taco
Chicken Fajita Pita
Salads:
   Asian Chicken Salad
   Southwest Chicken Salad
   Chicken Club Salad
   Side Salad

Kentucky Fried Chicken

Tender Roast Chicken
   Sandwich, no sauce
Honey BBQ Chicken Sandwich
Sides:
   Corn on the Cob
   BBQ Beans
   Green Beans

Long John Silver's

Chicken Sandwich
Sides:
   Corn Cobbette
   Rice

McDonald's

Breakfast:
   Low-Fat Apple Bran Muffin
   Scrambled Eggs
Chicken McGrill, no mayo
Hamburger
Cheeseburger
Salads, no dressing:
   Grilled Chicken Salad
      Deluxe
   Grilled Chicken Caesar
      Salad
   Grilled Chicken California
      Cobb Salad
   California Cobb Salad
   Caesar Salad
   Garden Salad
Snack Size Fruit in Yogurt
   Parfait
Vanilla Reduced-Fat Ice
   Cream Cone

Pizza Hut

Veggie Lover's (all varieties of
   pizza), 1 slice

Subway

Breakfast:

   Ham and Egg Sandwich

   Western Egg Sandwich

6-inch subs, no dressing

   or mayo:

   Ham

   Honey Mustard Turkey

   Roast Beef

   Turkey Breast

   Turkey and Ham

   Veggie Delite

   Roasted Chicken Breast

   Subway Club

Deli Sandwiches:

   Ham Deli Style Sandwich

   Roast Beef Deli Style

     Sandwich

   Turkey Breast Deli Style

     Sandwich

Salads, no dressing:

   Ham Salad

   Roast Beef

   Roasted Chicken

     Breast

   Subway Club

   Tuna, light mayo

   Turkey Breast Salad

   Turkey Breast and Ham

   Veggie Delite Salad

Soups:

   Black Bean

Brown and Wild Rice with

   Chicken

Minestrone

New England Clam Chowder

Roasted Chicken Noodle

Tomato Bisque

Vegetable Beef

Taco Bell

Taco

Tostada

Soft Taco, Steak

Soft Taco, Light Chicken

Chicken Burrito, Light

Sides:

   Mexican Rice

Wendy's

Jr. Hamburger

Jr. Cheeseburger

Grilled Chicken Sandwich

Fresh Stuffed Pita—Caesar,

   Garden, or Chicken

Salad, no dressing:

   Caesar Side Salad

   Deluxe Garden Salad

   Grilled Chicken Salad

   Mandarin Chicken Salad

   Spring Mix Salad

   Side Salad

Baked Potato, Plain

Chili, Plain

Supplement D

Workout Diary

Use this diary to keep track of your exercise performance. Recording your progress, and seeing it in black and white, help boost your motivation. The sample entry provides an example of how to record your exercise activities and performance. Blank forms for your use are on the following pages.

Day of the Week	Time	Activity	Duration/Level of Effort
Sample	7 a.m.	Walking	30 minutes, 2 miles
(This shows you	5 p.m.	Weight training	Leg extensions: 30 lb,
how to log in		routine	12 reps; 40 lb, 10 reps
activities such as			Leg curls: 40 lb, 9 reps;
aerobics and			45 lb, 8 reps
weight training.			Sit-ups: 25 reps
So that you don't			Bench press: 10 lb,
overdo, it's best			12 reps; 15 lb, 8 reps
to do these on			Shoulder press: 10 lb,
separate days.)			12 reps; 15 lb, 10 reps
			Arm curls: 10 lb, 12 reps;
			15 lb, 8 reps

Day of the Week	Time	Activity	Duration/Level of Effort
Sunday			
Monday			
Tuesday			
Wednesday			
Thursday			

Day of the Week	Time	Activity	Duration/Level of Effort
Friday			
Saturday			

Day of the Week	Time	Activity	Duration/Level of Effort
Sunday			
Monday			
Tuesday			
Wednesday			
Thursday			

Day of the Week	Time	Activity	Duration/Level of Effort
Friday			
Saturday			

Day of the Week	Time	Activity	Duration/Level of Effort
Sunday			
Monday			
Tuesday			
Wednesday			
Thursday			

Day of the Week	Time	Activity	Duration/Level of Effort
Friday			
Saturday			

Supplement E

Resources

Anorexia Nervosa and Related Eating Disorders, Inc.
P.O. Box 5102
Eugene, OR
(800) 931-2237
(541) 344-1144
Website: www.anred.com

**National Association of Anorexia Nervosa
and Associated Disorders**
P.O. Box 7
Highland Park, IL 60035
(847) 831-3438
Website: www.anad.org

National Eating Disorders Association
603 Steward Street, Suite 803
Seattle, WA 98101
(206) 382-3587
Website: www.nationaleatingdisorders.org

About the Author

Jay McGraw is the teen expert on the *Dr. Phil* show. He is the author of the *New York Times* bestseller *Life Strategies for Teens,* and *Closing the Gap.* He is currently in law school at Southern Methodist University in Dallas, Texas. He enjoys spending time with his friends and his brother, Jordan.